HOME
DOCTOR

LONDON, NEW YORK, MUNICH, MELBOURNE, DELHI

US Senior Editor Jill Hamilton
US Editor Jane Perlmutter
US Editorial Assistant Madeline Farbman
UK Editors Esther Ripley, Alyson Lacewing, Dawn Henderson
Senior Managing Editor Martyn Page
Project Art Editors Sue Caws, Isabel de Cordova
DTP Designer Julian Dams
Managing Art Editor Marianne Markham
Picture Researchers Romaine Werblow, Claire Bowers, Juliet Duff, Carolyn Clerkin
Jacket Editor Beth Apple
Jacket Designer Natalie Godwin
Production Controller Louise Daly
Category Publishers Jackie Douglas, Mary Thompson, Corinne Roberts
Art Director Bryn Walls
Additional Design Inperspective Ltd., Ist Floor, Exmouth House, 3–11 Pine Street, London EC1R 0JH

Published in the US by DK Publishing, Inc.
375 Hudson Street, New York, New York 10014
First American Edition 2004

04 05 06 07 08 10 9 8 7 6 5 4 3 2 1

Every effort has been made to ensure that the information in this book is accurate. The information in this book will be relevant to the majority of people but may not be applicable in each individual case, so you are therefore advised to obtain expert medical advice for specific information on personal health matters. Never disregard expert medical advice or delay in receiving treatment due to information obtained from this book. The naming of any product, treatment, or organization in this book does not imply endorsement by the author or the publisher, nor does the omission of any such names indicate disapproval. Neither the publisher nor the author accept any legal responsibility for any personal injury or other damage or loss arising from any use or misuse of the information and advice in this book.

A Cataloging-in-Publication record for this book is available from the Library of Congress.
ISBN 0-7566-0347-1

Color reproduction by Colourscan, Singapore
Printed and bound in Singapore by Star Standard Industries (Pte.) Ltd.

HOME
DOCTOR

Dr. Michael Peters

US consultant editor

Adriane Fugh-Berman, M.D.

A Dorling Kindersley Book

Forewords

Dr. Peters has written a very useful, extensive home medical reference that contains a wealth of practical, easy-to-follow advice. Each condition is introduced with a short description, and circumstances under which one should consult a doctor immediately are conveniently placed first. For illnesses that can be safely treated at home, effective nonprescription treatments are recommended, as well as non-drug treatments such as peppermint oil for irritable bowel syndrome, feverfew to prevent migraines, and relaxation exercises for stress.

The major strength of this book lies in the hundreds of practical tips and techniques for treating – and preventing – common symptoms and illnesses. The illustrations are an excellent complement to the text and are very helpful for demonstrating, for example, the technique for steam inhalation, how to stop a nosebleed, or how to get out of bed when one has back pain. The techniques for calming a baby with sleep problems or colic will be quite valuable to new parents. First aid is also covered, and a glossary of nonprescription treatments mentioned in the book is included.

It is clear that Dr. Peters is a competent, experienced physician with loads of common sense. This book contains an enormous amount of practical, easily understood information, and would be an excellent addition to any home library.

Adriane Fugh-Berman, M.D.

People today are more aware of health issues than ever before, but they are frequently confronted with a bewildering array of self-help advice. There is often little guidance through this maze, leaving many confused about when and whom to ask for help, and sometimes suffering because they do not want to bother their doctor with "trivial" complaints.

As a general practitioner for many years, I have always felt it is important to empower people by giving them clear information to enable them to make sensible decisions about their health. In writing *Home Doctor* I have tried to put this into practice, covering over 150 common conditions for which home treatment is often appropriate. In each article, I have given guidance on identifying your condition and deciding whether self-help is suitable, and advised on practical help and treatment.

A range of drug and natural remedies is suggested in this book (with more information, such as brand names, listed in an A–Z list at the back). There is a vast number of treatments available in pharmacies and health stores, but I have confined myself to those that are likely to be most effective. Naturally, there will be omissions or alternatives that may be just as suitable. As much as possible, I have used a similar evidence-based approach in choosing natural remedies, with the occasional addition of a soothing herbal tea or oil that may help and is unlikely to cause harm.

In researching and writing this book, I have tried to create a simple home reference that can be turned to when any family member is sick or needs medical advice. However, a book can give only general guidance and is no substitute for professional advice. When you can't find an answer here, or are in any doubt about a medical condition, you should see your own doctor.

Michael Peters

Dr. Michael Peters

Contents

How to use this book

Home Doctor is divided into three main sections. The first, Common Conditions, is the core of the book, providing detailed advice on home treatment for a wide range of everyday disorders and complaints. The second section, First Aid, describes basic first-aid treatment for minor and more serious emergencies; and the final A–Z of Drug and Natural Remedies supplies further information on remedies suggested in articles.

Common Conditions

is divided into general symptoms; infectious diseases; groups of disorders such as eye and ear problems; and problems specific to men, women, children, and babies.

Summary of the symptoms of an illness and whom it affects helps you identify the problem

What you can do yourself advises on treatment. Icons direct you to Drug remedies, Natural remedies, and Practical technique and tips boxes

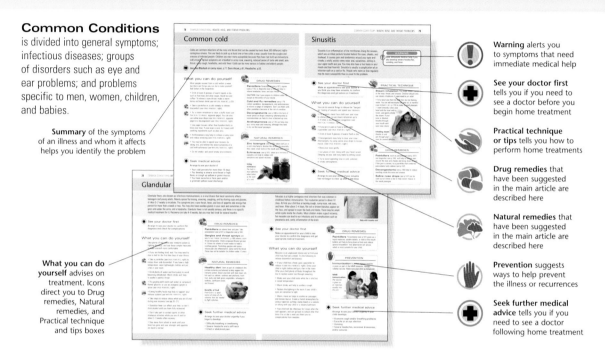

Warning alerts you to symptoms that need immediate medical help

See your doctor first tells you if you need to see a doctor before you begin home treatment

Practical technique or tips tells you how to perform home treatments

Drug remedies that have been suggested in the main article are described here

Natural remedies that have been suggested in the main article are described here

Prevention suggests ways to help prevent the illness or recurrences

Seek further medical advice tells you if you need to see a doctor following home treatment

First Aid

provides basic first-aid advice for minor mishaps and injuries, and step-by-step techniques to help you deal with serious injuries and emergencies.

Warning alerts you to when you need to call 911

Summary of the injury or emergency helps you decide how to act

Practical technique gives step-by-step instructions for emergency treatment

A–Z of Drug and Natural Remedies

gives information, such as brand names, side effects, and precautions, for the treatments suggested in articles and general advice on using them safely.

Drug remedy

Natural remedy

Each entry includes brand names, uses, method of use, side effects, and precautions

Symptom finder

Knowing exactly what is wrong when you are not feeling well is not always easy. Individual symptoms can be caused by a variety of different illnesses, and some disorders produce surprising effects on the body that seem unrelated to the initial problem. If you are unsure which article to consult, use this symptom finder as a starting point. Each symptom listed has page references that take you to the articles in which it is covered.

Symptom finder continued

COMMON CONDITIONS

This major part of the book features a wide

range of common illnesses and disorders that

can usually be treated successfully at home.

The first section, covering general symptoms,

such as fever or fatigue, that are common to

many illnesses, is followed by coverage of

the most prevalent infectious diseases.

Conditions are then organized according

to the parts of the body they affect,

such as the chest and abdomen,

or the eyes and ears. Specific

problems affecting men, women,

children, and babies are dealt

with in their own sections.

GENERAL SYMPTOMS

Fever

In a fever, your body temperature is raised persistently above the normal level of 98.6°F (37°C). A fever is one way in which the body responds to infection, so it is likely to result from a viral illness such as the flu, or a throat, chest, or bladder infection. It can also be due to other diseases, heatstroke, sunburn, or reactions to drugs. At first you feel warm; if your temperature continues to rise, you feel chilled and may shiver, then as it drops you feel hot and flushed. You may become dehydrated if a fever persists.

WARNING

Get medical help immediately if:
- Temperature is over 103°F (39.4°C)
- You have a headache, sensitivity to light, stiff neck, and/or a rash
- You are drowsy or confused
- You have difficulty breathing

 ## See your doctor first

Arrange to see your doctor promptly if you feel weak and very ill, and/or if you have a specific symptom with a fever, such as an earache, a rash, or a cough with phlegm.

DRUG REMEDIES

Analgesics such as acetaminophen (*see* p.177) and ibuprofen (*see* p.185) will reduce fever and help to relieve headache and muscle aches. Start taking an analgesic as soon as you begin to feel feverish.

What you can do yourself

Use the following measures in conjunction with any treatment from your doctor.

- Rest; you don't have to stay in bed, but don't overexert yourself. Don't go to work.

- Take an analgesic (*see* DRUG REMEDIES, right).

- Drink at least 8 glasses of water or diluted fruit juice to help prevent dehydration. Try to have 1 glass of fluid an hour. Avoid caffeinated drinks. Try soups and broths if you feel unable to eat.

- Keep cool, but avoid getting cold. Wear light, loose clothes. In hot weather, use an electric fan.

- To check your temperature, use a digital thermometer (*see* PRACTICAL TECHNIQUE, right).

- If you are shivering, don't try to warm yourself. Instead, cover yourself up with a sheet or with a light blanket.

- If you feel hot and sweaty, sponge your face with lukewarm water.

PRACTICAL TECHNIQUE

Checking your temperature Use a digital thermometer placed in your mouth or armpit, or an aural thermometer, the tip of which is inserted in the ear. Forehead temperature strips are not reliable.

Using a digital thermometer
Hold in place until it beeps, then read the temperature display.

 ## Seek further medical advice

Arrange to see your doctor if:

- Your temperature keeps rising despite attempts to bring it down
- The fever has not subsided within 2 days and/or you have developed other symptoms

Excessive sweating

Almost everyone sweats more than usual when exercising or in hot weather, but some people generally sweat too much. Excessive sweating is common in adolescence but can continue throughout life. It can cause body odor and affect work and social relationships. People who sweat excessively are also more prone to fungal skin infections. Although some people are naturally susceptible to this problem, other factors, such as stress and anxiety, may have a significant role. Excessive sweating sometimes occurs in women around the time of menopause, or as a feature of conditions such as an overactive thyroid gland.

 See also **Athlete's foot and jock itch,** p.44.

 ## See your doctor first

Make an appointment to see your doctor if:

- The sweating is prolonged or unusual
- You are losing weight

What you can do yourself

There are some useful home treatments that help reduce sweating and body odor.

- Bathe or shower at least once daily in warm (but not hot) water. Dry yourself thoroughly afterward.

  - Use an antiperspirant or an antiperspirant combined with a deodorant. If an ordinary product does not work, try a stronger preparation containing aluminum chloride (*see* DRUG REMEDIES, right).

- Wear clean underwear and clothes every day. Choose natural fabrics, such as cotton, particularly next to your skin. Avoid tight clothes.

- If your feet get sweaty, wear leather shoes and cotton socks, and change both regularly. Go barefoot or wear sandals whenever possible.

- Drink at least 8 glasses of water a day, to replace lost body fluids. Cut down on alcohol and drinks containing caffeine, particularly hot drinks.

- Avoid spicy foods, which are likely to make you sweat, and onions and garlic, because of the odor.

- If you sweat when you are anxious, try practical techniques that reduce stress (*see* pp.20–21).

- If you are overweight, try to lose some weight.

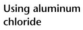 ### DRUG REMEDIES

Antiperspirants and deodorants
Antiperspirants block the pores that produce sweat, while deodorants attack the skin bacteria that cause body odor. Many products contain a combination of the two. Apply them daily after washing. If you develop skin irritation, use a hypoallergenic product. Absorbent, deodorizing foot powders are available for feet.

Aluminum chloride preparations
treat excessive sweating. Available as a roll-on applied to dry skin at nighttime. You can wash or shower the next day. One application can prevent sweating for 3 days or longer. Don't use on broken or irritated skin or near eyes, or if you have recently shaved or used depilatories.

Using aluminum chloride
Wash thoroughly and make sure that your skin is completely dry before you apply the antiperspirant.

 ## Seek further medical advice

Arrange to see your doctor if:

- You are still troubled by excessive sweating or body odor after following the advice described here
- You have any other symptoms associated with the excessive sweating

Itching

Itching is often a minor problem, but continual scratching may damage your skin and make the problem worse. A small area of itching may be caused by an insect bite or occur with a rash as a reaction to plants, metals, chemicals, or cosmetics. Larger areas may be due to dry skin, heat rash, hives, infections such as ringworm or scabies, or skin diseases such as eczema and psoriasis. Itching all over the body can be due to disorders such as diabetes, liver problems, or drug reactions. Stress and anxiety may cause or aggravate itching.

 See also Scabies, p.35; Urticaria, p.36; Eczema, p.38; Psoriasis, p.39; Dry skin, p.41; Heat rash, p.46; Ringworm, p.48; Insect bites and stings, p.158.

 See your doctor first

Consult your doctor if you think itching may be caused by a prescribed medicine.

What you can do yourself

There are several measures that you can take to help relieve itching.

- Try to resist scratching, and keep your fingernails short to limit any damage.

- Apply a cold compress. Soak a clean washcloth in cold water, wring it out, then place it on the itchy area. Repeat as necessary.

 - Apply a soothing preparation such as calamine lotion (*see* DRUG REMEDIES, right).

 - Try a mild hydrocortisone cream (*see* DRUG REMEDIES, right) for a localized area of red, itchy skin caused by an irritant, such as a cleaning product or metal jewelry. The cream is also helpful for insect bites and stings.

 - Take antihistamine pills to relieve itching that keeps you awake at night (*see* DRUG REMEDIES, right). Antihistamine cream can be used to relieve insect bites and stings.

- Moisturize and protect dry skin (*see* p.41).

- If stress aggravates itching, try some deep breathing exercises and muscle relaxation techniques (*see* PRACTICAL TECHNIQUES, pp.20–21).

- If possible, avoid hot or humid environments.

- Wear loose-fitting clothes made from natural fibers, but avoid wearing wool next to your skin.

DRUG REMEDIES

Calamine lotion (*see* p.179) has a cooling and soothing effect on irritated skin. You can apply calamine lotion to itchy areas as often as you need to. Dab it on with cotton balls and let it dry.

Hydrocortisone cream (*see* p.184) reduces itching and redness and is useful for treating allergic skin reactions and insect stings. Don't use it on children under 2 without medical advice.

Antihistamines (*see* p.178) such as diphenhydramine can be taken orally to relieve itching. They make you feel drowsy, so they will also help you sleep.

PREVENTION

Avoiding triggers for itching Once itching is under control, try to identify what causes it or makes it worse, if this isn't already obvious.

- Keep a diary, noting when you feel itchy and which products you use on your skin or clothing. If you suspect itching is due to a skin product, switch to a mild, unperfumed brand. If the cause is a laundry soap, use a nonallergenic one and an extra rinse.

 Seek further medical advice

Arrange to see your doctor if:

- Itching does not subside after about a week
- You develop other symptoms, such as jaundice or weight loss

Fatigue

Everyone feels tired after physical exertion or long periods of hard work. A good night's sleep usually solves the problem, but sometimes fatigue seems to drag on for days, and can interfere with your daily activities. The most obvious cause is difficulty sleeping, but you may also feel tired if you are stressed, a bit depressed, or if you've recently suffered a bereavement. An unhealthy diet and lack of exercise are common contributory factors. Viral illnesses such as mononucleosis and the flu can leave you tired for weeks afterward. Sometimes, persistent fatigue is due to an underlying condition such as anemia or a thyroid problem.

 See also **Difficulty sleeping**, p.17; **Stress**, pp.20–21; **Feeling depressed**, pp.22–23.

 ## See your doctor first

Make an appointment to see your doctor if:

- Fatigue is persistent and sleep doesn't help
- You often feel tired for no apparent reason

What you can do yourself

If you feel tired all the time, try the following adjustments to help you get your energy back.

- Even when you're very busy, get enough sleep each night. Overdoing things, then trying to catch up on your rest at the weekends, will disturb your sleep routine and leave you even more tired.

- Never miss breakfast. Include fresh vegetables, fruit, cereals, whole-grain bread and pasta, and brown rice in your diet. Cut down on fatty foods, such as cheese and red meat, and on sugar and salt.

- Check that you are not overweight or too thin. If you need to lose or gain weight, do so gradually.

- Try to spend time each day in fresh air. Exercise regularly, particularly if you have a sedentary job.

 - If you are sleepy during the day or while driving, try a "power nap" (*see* PRACTICAL TECHNIQUE, right).

- If you have had a viral illness, such as the flu or mononucleosis, it may be weeks before you're back to normal. Take time off to recover and take things easy when you return to work or school.

- If stress is contributing to "burnout," make more time for leisure activities. Try some deep breathing and muscle relaxation exercises (*see* PRACTICAL TECHNIQUES, pp.20–21).

PRACTICAL TECHNIQUE

Power napping If you find yourself nodding off during the day or you feel drowsy while driving, a brief nap may help you function better.

- An ideal nap lasts about 10–15 minutes, but even a 5-minute nap will leave you brighter and sharper afterward. Sleeping for more than 15 minutes helps, but you may feel groggy afterward. More than 30 minutes may affect your ability to sleep at night.
- Take a daily nap at the same time each day so your body gets used to the routine. Use an alarm clock or watch if you are worried about sleeping for too long.
- Don't nap late in the day or fall asleep in front of the TV in the evening, and don't use naps to catch up on sleep if you are having difficulty sleeping.

Timed nap
Set a watch or clock to wake you from your nap after about 15 minutes.

 ## Seek further medical advice

Arrange to see your doctor if:

- You still feel tired after trying these measures for 2–3 weeks, or you develop other symptoms

Hangover

A hangover is usually the result of drinking too much alcohol, but some people have symptoms after just a small amount of alcohol. The cause is a combination of the dehydrating effects of alcohol and adverse reactions to chemical additives in drinks, particularly dark-colored drinks such as red wine, port, brandy, and sherry. You may have a headache, nausea, dizziness, a dry mouth, and a raging thirst, which may disturb your sleep at night. Most people recover rapidly with some self-help measures.

 See also **Headache**, p.85; **Nausea and vomiting**, p.109.

What you can do yourself

If you know you have drunk too much, take the following steps immediately to minimize a hangover. Most symptoms clear up within 24 hours.

 ● Drink plenty of nonalcoholic fluids before going to bed and the next morning to reduce dehydration. Have a glass of water by your bed, and take sips if you wake up in the night. Fruit juices, which contain the natural sugar fructose, are particularly helpful (*see* NATURAL REMEDIES, right). Don't drink tea or coffee because they irritate the stomach and increase dehydration.

● Eat if you can. Even a banana will help boost low blood sugar levels.

 ● Take an analgesic to help prevent or relieve a headache (*see* DRUG REMEDIES, right).

 ● An antacid will help reduce nausea (*see* DRUG REMEDIES, right).

● Don't drink more alcohol to reduce your symptoms; this will only prolong the hangover.

● Rest until you begin to feel better.

● Don't drive. Alcohol remains in the bloodstream for long periods, so your reflexes may still be impaired the day after you have been drinking.

Seek medical advice

Arrange to see your doctor if:

● You have regular hangovers and are finding it hard to reduce your drinking
● You feel the need to drink alcohol first thing in the morning

---

NATURAL REMEDIES

Fructose is a natural sugar that can help the body to burn up alcohol faster. Plenty of fruit, juices, and honey will help you recover from a hangover.

Source of fructose
Eat an orange or drink some freshly squeezed juice to speed recovery.

DRUG REMEDIES

Analgesics such as ibuprofen (*see* p.185) or acetaminophen (*see* p.177) will help relieve a headache. Taking ibuprofen before you go to sleep may actually prevent some of the symptoms of a hangover (although it may worsen any stomach irritation).

Antacids (*see* p.177) work by neutralizing stomach acids that contribute to nausea and indigestion. Antacids come in soothing liquids, carbonated drinks, and hard or chewable pills (chewing well before swallowing will allow them to work faster and increase their effectiveness).

PREVENTION

Avoiding a hangover If you know you are going to drink alcohol, try the following steps.

● Eat a meal before you start drinking.
● Alternate between alcoholic and soft drinks.

Difficulty sleeping

Many people have difficulty sleeping, either because they find it hard to get to sleep at night or because they wake early and cannot get back to sleep. Adults need 7–8 hours of sleep, on average, but people need less as they get older, and elderly people may need as little as 5–6 hours. An occasional sleepless night won't do you any harm, although you may feel tired the next day. More persistent sleep disturbances are often due to stress, anxiety, or depression and may leave you continually tired, irritable, and unable to concentrate. Physical symptoms such as pain, breathing problems, and hot flashes, and some medicines, can also disturb sleep.

 See also **Stress**, pp.20–21; **Feeling depressed**, pp.22–23.

See your doctor first

Make an appointment to see your doctor if:

- You feel depressed
- Physical symptoms are preventing sleep

What you can do yourself

There are several things you can try to make it easier to get a good night's sleep.

- Go to bed and get up at the same times each day. Even if you are tired, don't take naps during the day.

- Don't eat a heavy or rich meal less than 3 hours before you go to bed. Avoid coffee, tea, cola, alcohol, and smoking. If you are hungry, eat a cookie or a banana. Drink a glass of warm milk half an hour before bedtime.

 - Use practical measures to help you get over your sleep difficulties (*see* PRACTICAL TIPS, right).

 - Try an herbal remedy that promotes sleep (*see* NATURAL REMEDIES, right).

 - If you're feeling tense, practice relaxation exercises (*see* pp.20–21) shortly before bedtime. Soak in a warm bath. Lavender oil (*see* NATURAL REMEDIES, right) may be helpful.

 - Taking a sedative antihistamine may relieve a temporary sleep problem (*see* DRUG REMEDIES, right).

Seek further medical advice

Arrange to see your doctor if you still cannot sleep after trying the measures given above.

PRACTICAL TIPS

Managing sleeplessness Try these tips, and keep using them until they begin to work.

- Stop working at least an hour before bedtime and read a book or listen to relaxing music. Keep your bedroom quiet, dark, and not too hot or cold.
- If you can't fall asleep within 30 minutes, get up, go into another room, and read. Don't watch TV.
- If your head is buzzing with tasks for the next day, keep a notepad by your bed and jot them down.

NATURAL REMEDIES

Herbal sleeping remedies (*see* p.184) Tinctures or pills containing valerian, passionflower, or hops may help promote restful sleep.

Lavender oil (*see* p.185) is a traditional sleep remedy. Try inhaling it, or adding it to a warm bath before bedtime.

Using lavender
Try putting a bag of dried lavender or some drops of lavender oil on a tissue inside your pillowcase.

DRUG REMEDIES

Antihistamines (*see* p.178) Sedative types are useful for treating short-term insomnia.

Jet lag

Jet lag is a collection of symptoms that occur while your body clock adjusts to a new time zone when you travel. Until you get used to the local time, you may feel disoriented and tired during the day and have difficulty sleeping at the new nighttime. You may also experience poor concentration, loss of appetite, and diarrhea or constipation. Most people begin to feel the effects of jet lag only after crossing three or more time zones. Traveling from east to west (for example, from London to New York) extends the day and is usually easier on the body than traveling from west to east, which shortens the day. People tend to become more susceptible to the effects of jet lag as they get older.

What you can do yourself

Although jet lag usually lasts no more than a few days, use these tips to reduce its effects and adjust quickly to the new time zone.

- If possible, fly during the day. You are less likely to feel jet lag if you arrive at your destination in the evening and then stay awake until bedtime.

- Get plenty of rest before you depart: at least 8 hours' sleep a night in the week before you travel.

- Start adjusting to the new time zone when you begin your journey (*see* PRACTICAL TIPS, right).

- Drink plenty of water or fruit juice before and during the flight to prevent dehydration, and avoid alcohol, coffee, or cola drinks. Eat light meals and avoid fatty or salty foods.

- As soon as you arrive at your destination, adopt the local eating, waking, and sleeping times. Take a walk in daylight to help your body clock adjust.

- Avoid alcohol or caffeinated drinks within 3 hours of bedtime since they will make sleep more difficult.

- Jet lag can affect judgment and concentration, so do not drive until you have adapted to local time.

- If you travel frequently, try using antihistamine pills to relieve temporary sleep disturbances (*see* DRUG REMEDIES, right). Alternatively, ask your doctor for a short-acting prescription sleeping pill.

- If you are spending less than 2 days in a new time zone, you may be better off getting up, eating, and sleeping according to your home time.

- Seek your doctor's advice before traveling if you have to take prescribed medicines, such as insulin or birth control pills, at specific times of the day.

PRACTICAL TIPS

Adjusting to time zones Get used to the new time zone by setting your watch to your destination time as soon as you board the plane. If possible, plan your meals and sleep times around this time during the flight.

- If you need to sleep on the flight, listen to soft music, use earplugs, wear a sleep mask, and use a neck pillow.
- If you need to stay awake, keep active: get up and walk around the plane every hour, talk to your neighbor, read, or watch the in-flight entertainment.

DRUG REMEDIES

Antihistamines Sedative antihistamines (*see* p.178) cause drowsiness and can be used for a few days to help you reestablish your normal sleeping pattern. They are not addictive. Ask your pharmacist for advice on an appropriate type.

 Seek medical advice

Arrange to see your doctor if:

- **You are still experiencing symptoms of jet lag 2 weeks after traveling**

Feeling dizzy or faint

Dizzy spells and feeling faint are common problems. Causes include low blood sugar, drinking too much alcohol, or simply getting up too quickly. Feeling faint may also be due to emotional shock or panic, or may occur in pregnancy. An occasional episode is rarely a cause for concern, but sometimes the problem is due to an underlying condition or to certain drugs.

See also Panic attacks, p.24.

WARNING

Seek immediate medical help if you are dizzy or faint and have:

- Diabetes
- Chest pain or palpitations
- Weakness in your arms or legs, slurred speech, or blurred vision

See your doctor first

Make an appointment to see your doctor if:

- You are taking a prescribed medicine that may be causing the problem, such as drugs for high blood pressure or tranquilizers

What you can do yourself

There are several things you can do to help yourself get over fainting a or dizzy spell quickly.

- Keep your head down on your knees or your feet raised and take deep breaths (*see* PRACTICAL TECHNIQUE, right).

- If it has been several hours since you last ate, eat or drink a snack that contains sugar (not something containing artificial sweeteners).

- Don't drink caffeinated drinks such as coffee, tea, cola, or alcohol, and don't smoke, since all of these can make your symptoms worse.

- Don't try to drive or operate machinery until you are completely recovered.

Seek further medical advice

Arrange to see your doctor if:

- You do not recover promptly from an episode of dizziness or feeling faint
- You have repeated episodes of feeling faint or dizzy, or you develop any other symptoms

PRACTICAL TECHNIQUE

Recovery measures If you feel faint or dizzy, sit down and put your head on your knees. Alternatively, lie down and raise your legs on a chair or cushion. Try to keep calm, because fast breathing (hyperventilating) and anxiety can make symptoms worse. Breathe slowly and deeply. Open a window or go out into fresh air if you feel steady on your feet.

Helping blood flow
Lean forward and put your head down to improve the blood flow to your brain.

PREVENTION

Avoiding dizzy spells Combine these steps with any treatment from your doctor to help prevent further attacks.

- Avoid hot and stuffy environments. Have a window open, or go out into fresh air from time to time.
- Don't get up suddenly after lying down or sitting.
- Drink at least 6–8 glasses of water a day.
- Eat regularly. Have healthy snacks, such as fruit, between meals to keep your blood sugar level steady.
- Avoid straining on the toilet, since this can cause a drop in blood pressure and make you feel faint.
- If you are pregnant, don't stand for long periods or lie flat on your back.

Stress

When you are under stress, your muscles tighten, your heart beats faster, your breathing becomes rapid and shallow, and your brain becomes more alert. In small doses, stress can improve your performance in situations such as sports activities or work, but if excessive or prolonged it can harm your health. You may suffer from poor appetite, headaches, migraines, difficulty sleeping, and increased susceptibility to infections. You may also feel anxious, irritable, unable to concentrate, tired, sad, or depressed. Stress tends to build up when the normal pressures of life become too much for you, or may be triggered by an upsetting event such as a death.

 See also **Fatigue**, p.15; **Difficulty sleeping**, p.17; **Feeling depressed**, pp.22–23; **Panic attacks**, p.24.

What you can do yourself

People react differently to stress depending on their personality and the support they have around them. Although you can't always control difficult events in your life, you can adapt the way in which you react to everyday stresses and learn how to avoid some of them.

● Get adequate sleep; if you are tired you are more likely to feel stressed.

● Eat regularly to keep your energy levels constant during the day. Never miss breakfast. Include fresh fruit, cereal, whole-grain bread, pasta, and rice in your diet. Cut down on foods such as cheese, eggs, red meat, and butter that are high in fat. Reduce your intake of sugar and salt.

● Cut down on or cut out caffeine by limiting your intake of coffee, tea, cola, and chocolate.

● Get regular exercise, especially if you have a sedentary job. Exercise produces "feel-good" chemicals in the brain that increase your sense of well-being. Try 15–30 minutes of brisk walking, or go swimming or bicycling.

● Set aside a regular time each day specifically for relaxation: do not wait until you feel exhausted. Go for a regular walk; listen to music; or try meditation or yoga.

● Imagine that you are in a place where you feel warm, relaxed, and comfortable, such as lying on a sunny beach. Try to imagine all the colors, sounds, smells, and feelings.

 ● Practice deep, controlled breathing with exercises that can be used whenever you feel tense (*see* PRACTICAL TECHNIQUE, right).

 PRACTICAL TECHNIQUE

Deep breathing This exercise helps calm your body and mind. Deep breathing using the diaphragm and abdominal muscles is the basis of most relaxation methods. Find a place where you won't be interrupted, take the phone off the hook and/or switch off your cell phone, and practice these exercises for 10–20 minutes each day.

1 *Wear loose clothing and sit or lie in a comfortable position. Place one hand on your chest and the other on your abdomen. Breathe in slowly through your nose, hold your breath for a moment, then breathe out slowly. Try to breathe using your abdominal muscles so the lower hand moves more than the upper one.*

2 *Once you know that you are breathing from your abdomen, place your hands just below your ribs. Feel your hands move as your abdomen rises and falls. When you feel more relaxed, let your hands drop down by your sides and simply enjoy the relaxation.*

What you can do yourself *continued...*

- When you are in the middle of a stressful situation, try to have a few minutes alone. Go for a brisk walk or sit somewhere quiet to help you relax.

- If your muscles have become tense, try to relax them regularly (*see* PRACTICAL TECHNIQUE, right).

- Try to control self-criticism. To counteract it, remind yourself of your good points and the successes you have had in the past.

- Don't bottle up your worries; it usually helps to share problems with family members and friends.

- Don't try a short-term "fix" by turning to alcohol or illegal drugs. In the long term they will only add to your problems.

✚ Seek medical advice

Arrange to see your doctor if:

- You feel unable to cope with stress
- You feel depressed

PREVENTION

Limiting stress If you have a great deal of stress in your life, the following steps will help you deal with it and feel healthier as a result.

- Over 2–3 weeks, make a note of the situations in which you felt under stress and whether stress made you perform better or worse than normal. Think about how you might have responded differently to feel more in control. Ask people close to you how they react in similar situations.
- Accept that there are some things you can't control, such as traffic delays on the way to work.
- Organize and prioritize your time. Do what is important first. Anticipate deadlines and reduce your other commitments around these times.
- Identify tasks and break them into smaller sections if they seem too big to manage all at once. Use a checklist and check off tasks as you complete them.
- Have realistic expectations. Don't commit yourself to tasks that you feel unable to do or don't want to do; delegate when you are able to do so. Don't feel demoralized or guilty if things go wrong.
- Take regular breaks throughout the day, even if it is only to look out the window. Have lunch breaks.

PRACTICAL TECHNIQUE

Relaxing muscles Learn to recognize when your muscles are tense, since this will help you control stress reactions. This exercise will enable you to relax problem areas consciously. If time is short, it may help to use the exercise on just one group of muscles, such as your shoulders. Keep your eyes closed throughout, and breathe slowly using your abdominal muscles (*see* opposite page).

1 *To prepare for the exercise, be aware of how your muscles feel in their relaxed state and when they are tense. Try to imagine the tension fading away as you relax each muscle.*

2 *Yawn, then relax. Clench your jaw, and release. Frown, scrunch up your eyes and nose, then let go. Raise your eyebrows, then relax all the muscles in your face.*

3 *Lift your shoulders up to your ears. Hold for a few seconds, then lower again. Repeat 2–3 times. To free the neck muscles, rock your head gently from side to side.*

4 *Tense and relax your stomach muscles, then each buttock in turn. Clench and release your right fist, then all the muscles in your arm. Repeat the process with your left arm.*

5 *Tense the muscles in your right foot, hold for a few seconds, then release. Tense and release the calf, then the thigh muscles. Repeat the process with the left foot and leg.*

Feeling depressed

Most people have occasional low moods, but if you are depressed they become persistent. You may feel tearful and low, particularly in the morning; lack energy and confidence; and find it hard to concentrate or make decisions. Sleep problems and loss of sex drive and appetite are common. Depression is often a reaction to a life event such as bereavement, or it may have no obvious cause. Lack of sunlight in winter makes some people feel sad, and 1 woman in 10 has depression after childbirth.

WARNING

Seek immediate medical help if:
- You are having suicidal thoughts
- You have recently had a baby and are having thoughts of harming yourself or your child

 See also **Stress**, pp.20–21.

 ## See your doctor first

Make an appointment to see your doctor if you have feelings of depression that last longer than a week.

What you can do yourself

There are several lifestyle changes and home treatments that can help you through a short period of feeling low. They will also support treatment given by your doctor.

- When you are depressed, even simple tasks may seem difficult. Set a small, achievable, pleasant goal for yourself each day, such as taking a walk around the block or having a special breakfast. Adopt the same approach if you feel you have an overwhelming list of problems. Tackle only one problem at a time; if necessary, break it down into smaller, achievable goals and work through them.

- If you have occasional sad or negative thoughts, distract yourself by listening to the radio or watching TV, which require little concentration.

- Try to avoid extra stress. If possible, postpone or delegate important decisions. Look rationally at the work you have to do; focus on essential tasks and sideline less important ones.

- Don't bottle things up. You may find it a relief to share your feelings and emotions with sympathetic relatives or close friends. Talking about problems is not a sign of weakness.

 ## NATURAL REMEDIES

St. John's wort (*see* p.189) is a popular herbal remedy for mild depression. Taken as a pill once a day, it appears to be as effective as some prescription antidepressants. Like prescribed drugs, it can take some time to work.

CAUTION: Check with your doctor first. Don't use St. John's wort if you are taking oral contraceptives, prescribed antidepressants, or any daily medication.

Essential fatty acids (*see* p.182), or EFAs, are obtained from foods and play an important part in forming healthy cells and nerve tissue. A group called omega-3 EFAs may also help regulate hormones and brain chemicals that control mood, and can help reduce symptoms of depression. You can boost levels of these EFAs by eating olive oil, walnuts, and oily fish, such as salmon and mackerel.

Boosting omega-3 EFAs
Make sure your diet includes 2 or 3 portions a week of oily fish, such as grilled salmon.

What you can do yourself *continued...*

- Try to eat regularly, even though you may not feel like it. Choose foods that you enjoy, but make sure you include plenty of vegetables, fruit, bread, pasta, rice, and potatoes. Have small portions if you don't feel like eating large meals.

- Exercise helps you relax, improves sleep, and may reduce depression by releasing chemicals in the brain that improve mood. Just going for a walk or doing some gardening is beneficial. Everybody should be capable of getting some exercise, but if you have a medical condition (such as arthritis or a heart problem), check with your doctor first.

 - Try the natural remedy St. John's wort to relieve low moods (*see* NATURAL REMEDIES, left).

 - Include foods such as oily fish and olive oil in your diet to boost your levels of essential fatty acids, or EFAs (*see* NATURAL REMEDIES, left). These substances may help combat depression.

- Cut down or stop drinking alcohol. Although it may appear to offer a "quick fix," alcohol can contribute to depression and also affects your physical health.

- Stop using any recreational drugs, such as marijuana or ecstasy; they can have long-term effects that contribute to depression.

- If your sleep is disturbed, try reducing your caffeine intake, and avoid sleeping in the day (*see* DIFFICULTY SLEEPING, p.17).

- If you regularly feel tense and find it difficult to unwind, try practicing deep breathing exercises and muscle relaxation methods (*see* PRACTICAL TECHNIQUES, pp.20–21).

- If possible, try to identify the cause of your depression. Defining your problem may help you stop feeling guilty about your feelings and, with time, you may become able to deal with the underlying difficulty.

 - If you are regularly depressed in the winter months (a condition known as seasonal affective disorder, or SAD) you may benefit from light treatment (*see* PRACTICAL TIPS, right).

PRACTICAL TIPS

Coping with SAD Symptoms of seasonal affective disorder usually develop as the days get shorter in the fall. You may feel sad, low, and tired, want to sleep more than you normally do, and have cravings for starchy or sugary foods. Increased exposure to natural light is thought to help SAD sufferers, so try the following tips.

- Try to get outdoors as much as possible on winter days. Even on dull, cloudy days you will benefit from exposure to natural light.
- Arrange work and home conditions so that you are exposed to as much natural light as possible. Work by a window if you can. Trim back trees and bushes around your home to let in light.
- If possible, treat yourself to a short winter break in a sunny area of the country.
- Some people find light therapy helpful. This is usually given using a special light box that emits a very bright light. Other devices simulate a natural dawn in the morning. Light boxes are usually expensive, so discuss what might be of value with your doctor before you invest in equipment.

Using light therapy
You can carry out normal activities, such as reading, working, or eating, while staying close to the light box.

 ### Seek further medical advice

Arrange to see your doctor if:

- **Your depression is becoming more severe and/or lasts longer than 2 weeks**
- **You are taking prescribed antidepressant drugs and they are not having an effect within the timespan suggested by your doctor**

Panic attacks

Panic attacks are episodes of intense fear with unpleasant physical symptoms that usually occur without any outside threat being present. You may be short of breath or breathe rapidly (hyperventilate) and suffer from sweating, dizziness, nausea, numbness, chest pains, or palpitations. Attacks may be linked to anxiety, stress, depression, a phobia (such as fear of flying), or taking stimulants or drugs, but symptoms can develop for no apparent reason. Although the attacks usually pass quickly, fear of having them can interfere with normal life.

 See also Stress, pp.20–21; **Feeling depressed**, pp.22–23; **Palpitations**, p.105.

 ### See your doctor first

Make an appointment to see your doctor to check that your symptoms aren't due to a more serious illness such as heart disease.

What you can do yourself

Take the following steps to calm yourself quickly and help you cope with future attacks.

- If you are hyperventilating, try rebreathing into a bag (*see* PRACTICAL TECHNIQUE, right).

- When you feel symptoms developing, focus steadily on something happening near you or on what someone else is saying, rather than concentrating on your own feelings. Remind yourself that, although your symptoms are unpleasant, they cannot harm you and will pass.

- Try not to avoid situations in which you are prone to attacks. If you start to confront them, your symptoms should begin to fade and you will begin to regain your confidence.

 ### Seek further medical advice

Arrange to see your doctor if:

- The above measures do not help
- Your panic attacks are becoming more frequent and/or are interfering with your life

 ## PRACTICAL TECHNIQUE

Rebreathing into a paper bag

Rapid breathing during a panic attack lowers carbon dioxide levels in your blood, making you feel dizzy and faint. Rebreathing from a paper bag, held loosely over your mouth and nose, will help restore carbon dioxide levels. Cup your hands over your mouth and nose if you don't have a bag.

Using a paper bag
Breathe in and out into the bag about 10 times, then breathe normally for 15 seconds. Continue until your breathing slows down.

 ## PREVENTION

Preventing panic attacks The following lifestyle changes and techniques can help prevent or at least minimize panic attacks.

- Practice deep breathing and muscle relaxation exercises (*see* PRACTICAL TECHNIQUES, pp.20–21) and use them whenever an attack is about to begin.
- Too much caffeine may trigger attacks, so reduce your intake of caffeinated drinks. Cut down on alcohol and smoking and don't take recreational drugs.
- Eat regular meals to keep blood sugar levels stable and prevent symptoms such as lightheadedness.
- Exercise regularly to boost general well-being.

Poor memory

Most people suffer from occasional forgetfulness, especially in later life when slower brain processing may make it harder for them to store and remember information. However, absentmindedness is not an inevitable part of aging, nor is it confined to the elderly. Poor memory can also be due to lack of sleep; an underlying condition such as depression; stress; a thyroid disorder; excessive use of alcohol; or prescribed or recreational drugs. In most cases, memory improves again when the underlying problem is treated. There are also techniques that help protect and sharpen memory skills at any age. When memory deterioration occurs with symptoms such as confusion, intellectual decline, and a change in personality, it may be a sign of dementia.

 ## See your doctor first

Make an appointment to see your doctor if:

- Your memory is deteriorating
- You are taking medication such as sleeping pills that may be affecting your memory

What you can do yourself

There are no instant cures for forgetfulness, but the following techniques and lifestyle changes can help preserve and improve your memory.

- Get a good night's sleep, get regular exercise, and include plenty of fresh fruits (especially citrus fruits), green leafy vegetables, nuts, olives, whole-grain bread, and cereals in your diet.

- Try not to worry about your memory failures; anxiety and lack of confidence will only make them worse. Figure out why you forgot something and organize yourself so it is less likely to happen again.

- Try techniques to improve your memory (*see* PRACTICAL TECHNIQUES, right). Exercise your brain with word games. Read rather than watch TV.

- Note tasks and events on a calendar and in a journal that you keep with you at all times. Be orderly: keep essential articles in their own place, such as keys and glasses by the front door. Have fixed days and times for important tasks.

- Don't drink excessively or take recreational drugs such as marijuana and ecstasy. However, drinking 1–2 ounces of alcohol a day (a glass of wine contains one ounce of alcohol) may help reduce the risk of dementia.

- Have your vision and hearing checked regularly.

PRACTICAL TECHNIQUES

Memory aids Most of the following techniques use visualization and repetition, which help store information in memory.

- Pay attention, particularly in situations where you feel excited or under stress. Ask people to repeat information that doesn't register immediately. Then repeat it in your own words. Note landmarks along your route in unfamiliar surroundings, such as a large building or driving through a new town.
- If you tend to forget a person's name moments after you are introduced, repeat the name back, then try to make a picture from it incorporating the person in front of you. For example, visualize Glenda Fisher fishing by a stream near a leafy glen.
- To remember a list, use a set of locations in your home and put an item from the list in each one. Make the mental images incongruous and exaggerated. For example, to remember a shopping list you could visualize a huge block of butter melting on your bed; a loaf of bread baking in the fireplace; or a giant tea bag in the sink. To recall the list in the supermarket, visualize walking through your home and finding each item in its strange location.
- Exercise your memory. Keep track of your money by remembering how and where you spent it since you last went to the bank. Alternatively, try to recall the main points of a recent conversation with a friend.

 ## Seek further medical advice

Arrange to see your doctor if:

- Your memory is continuing to decline and/or you are finding it difficult to cope

INFECTIOUS DISEASES

Mumps

Mumps is a viral infection that was common in children before routine immunization. The incubation period is 2–3 weeks. The illness usually starts with a fever, headache, and muscle aches. These are usually followed by swelling on one or both sides of the face and neck of the parotid salivary glands, which are just in front of and below the ears. Talking, eating, and drinking may be painful. Mumps is usually mild in children, but teenagers and adults may develop potentially serious complications.

> ## WARNING
>
> Contact your doctor urgently if any of the following develop:
> - Severe headache and avoidance of bright light
> - Vomiting, seizures, or excessive drowsiness

See your doctor first

Make an appointment to see your doctor to confirm mumps and check for complications.

What you can do yourself

There is no specific treatment for mumps, but you can make yourself or your child more comfortable.

- Rest until symptoms begin to ease.

- A warm compress, such as a washcloth soaked in warm water, applied to the side of the face, can help relieve pain in swollen glands.

- Drink plenty of fluids, but avoid acidic fruit juices because they stimulate saliva and may make the enlarged glands more painful. Use a straw if opening your mouth is painful.

- Have soup, yogurt, and other soft, bland foods that are easy to swallow.

- An analgesic will help reduce fever and relieve aches and pains (*see* DRUG REMEDIES, right).

- If mumps affects the testes, stay in bed and wear supportive clothing, such as two pairs of close-fitting underpants, until symptoms ease.

- If there are no complications, a child can usually go back to school, or an adult return to work, 5 days after the onset of the illness. Full recovery, however, can take 1–2 weeks.

> ## DRUG REMEDIES
>
> **Analgesics** will bring down a fever and relieve muscle aches and the pain of swollen glands.
>
> - For a child, give acetaminophen (*see* p.177), available as liquid medicine or chewable pills, or ibuprofen (*see* p.185), available as liquid medicine. Make sure you ask your pharmacist to recommend an appropriate product for your child.
> - Adults can take acetaminophen (*see* p.177) or ibuprofen (*see* p.185).

> ## PREVENTION
>
> **Immunization** to protect against mumps is given as part of the MMR (measles, mumps, rubella) vaccine. Make sure your child is immunized.

Seek further medical advice

Arrange to see your doctor if you or your child develops:

- Pain in the abdomen or chest
- Swelling and pain in the testes

Rubella

Rubella (German measles) is a contagious viral illness that is now uncommon due to immunization. Usually, it causes little more than a mild red rash that spreads from the face to the body. Often there are no symptoms. A child may start with a mild fever, swollen glands, and a runny nose 2–3 weeks after contact with the infection. Adults may also have a headache and joint pain. The main risk of rubella is that it can harm the fetus if a woman contracts the virus in pregnancy, particularly in the early months.

WARNING

Contact your doctor immediately if:

● You are pregnant and suspect you may have been in contact with someone who has rubella

 ## See your doctor first

Arrange to see your doctor if you suspect that you have rubella. Check when to attend the office, because of the risk of infecting a woman who is pregnant.

What you can do yourself

When there are symptoms, they are often so mild they need little or no treatment. The rash does not itch and disappears within a few days.

● Take an analgesic to reduce fever and relieve headache and joint pain (*see* DRUG REMEDIES, right).

● Drink plenty of fluids to prevent dehydration.

● As soon as you think that you have rubella, avoid contact with anyone who might be pregnant. Rubella is infectious for about 7 days before the rash develops and for about 5 days afterward.

 ## Seek further medical advice

Arrange to see your doctor if you develop:

● Headache or drowsiness
● Joint pain or sore eyes

DRUG REMEDIES

Analgesics will help bring down a fever and relieve headache and joint pain.

● For a child, give acetaminophen (*see* p.177) or ibuprofen (*see* p.185). Make sure you ask your pharmacist to recommend a product for your child.
● Adults can take acetaminophen (*see* p.177) or ibuprofen (*see* p.185).

PREVENTION

Immunization against rubella is given as part of the MMR (measles, mumps, rubella) vaccine.

● Make sure your child has the full recommended series of MMR immunizations.
● An attack of rubella also confers immunity, but if you plan to become pregnant, have your immunity checked first, even if you have had rubella. Make sure you are immunized, if necessary, before you conceive.

Immunity check
A simple blood test will establish your immunity to rubella.

Mononucleosis

Mononucleosis is a viral illness that most commonly affects teenagers and young adults. Mainly spread by kissing, sneezing, coughing, and by sharing cups and glasses, it takes 3–7 weeks to incubate. The symptoms are a sore throat, fever, and loss of appetite and energy that persist for more than a week or two. You may also have swollen glands in your neck and sometimes in your groin and under your arms, and a headache. Mononucleosis is not usually serious, and there is no specific medical treatment for it. Recovery can take 4–6 weeks, but you may feel tired for several months.

See your doctor first

Arrange to see your doctor to confirm the diagnosis and check for complications.

What you can do yourself

Get plenty of rest while your immune system is fighting the virus, and use these simple measures to make yourself more comfortable.

- If you are feeling tired, rest. You may need to stay in bed for the first few days of the illness.

- Take an analgesic (*see* DRUG REMEDIES, right) to reduce fever and discomfort. If you have a high temperature, wear lightweight clothes and put a fan in your room.

- Drink plenty of water and fruit juices to avoid becoming dehydrated. Warm drinks will help soothe a painful throat.

- Try gargling with warm salt water or you could use an analgesic gargle or spray (*see* DRUG REMEDIES, right).

- Eating healthy foods may help support your immune system (*see* NATURAL REMEDIES, right).

- Take steps to reduce stress while you are ill and during your recovery (*see* pp.20–21).

- Mononucleosis can affect your liver, so don't drink alcohol until you have fully recovered.

- Don't take part in contact sports or other strenuous activities while you are ill and for about 2–3 weeks after recovery.

- Stay away from school or work until your fever has gone and your strength and appetite are back to normal.

DRUG REMEDIES

Analgesics relieve fever and pain. Take acetaminophen (*see* p.177) or ibuprofen (*see* p.185).

Mouth and throat treatments (*see* p.187) can provide temporary relief from a sore throat. Dissolve a teaspoon of salt in a glass of warm water to make a soothing gargle. Lozenges containing benzocaine help numb a sore throat. Some mouth and throat treatments are not suitable for children; ask your pharmacist for advice.

NATURAL REMEDIES

Healthy diet Eaten as part of a balanced diet, certain nutrients are believed to help support the immune system. Boost your diet with lean meat; oily fish such as salmon, sardines, and herring; fresh fruit; leafy and dark green vegetables; wheat germ; walnuts; sunflower seeds; and flaxseed.

Benefits of fruit
Fresh fruit is a good source of many of the vitamins that are needed to fight infection.

Seek further medical advice

Arrange to see your doctor urgently if you begin to develop:

- Difficulty breathing or swallowing
- Severe headache and a stiff neck
- Chest or abdominal pain

Measles

Measles is a highly contagious viral infection that was common in children before immunization. The incubation period is about 10 days. At first your child has a hacking cough, runny nose, red eyes, and a fever. After about 2–4 days, flat red or brown blotches appear on the face, and spread to cover the body and limbs. There may be small white spots inside the cheeks. Most children make a good recovery, but measles can lead to ear infections and to complications such as pneumonia and, rarely, inflammation of the brain.

Child with measles rash

 ## See your doctor first

Make an appointment for your child to see your doctor to confirm the diagnosis and get appropriate medical treatment.

What you can do yourself

Measles is an unpleasant illness and at first your child may feel very unwell. Try the following to reduce discomfort and distress.

 ● If your child has a fever, give an analgesic to reduce it (*see* DRUG REMEDIES, right). Dress your child in light clothes and put a fan in the room. Offer your child plenty of fluids throughout the day to replace water lost through sweating.

● Although it is not necessary that your child stay in bed, it is necessary that he or she rest until the fever is gone.

● Warm drinks will help soothe a cough.

● Reduce the lighting in the room if your child's eyes are sensitive to light.

● Warm, moist air helps soothe air passages and loosen mucus. Create a humid atmosphere by using a vaporizer, putting a damp towel on a radiator, or sitting with your child in a steamy bathroom.

● Your child will be infectious for 5 days after the rash appears, and can go back to school after that time if he or she is well and there are no complications from measles.

 ### DRUG REMEDIES

Analgesics such as acetaminophen (*see* p.177), available as liquid medicine or chewable pills, or ibuprofen (*see* p.185), available as liquid medicine. Make sure you ask your pharmacist to recommend an appropriate product for your child.

 ### PREVENTION

Immunization to protect against measles is given as part of the MMR (measles, mumps, rubella) vaccine. Make sure your child is immunized.

MMR immunization
The vaccine is given as an injection, usually into the arm.

 ## Seek further medical advice

Arrange to see your doctor urgently if your child develops:

● A severe cough and/or breathing problems
● An earache or an eye infection
● Vomiting
● Severe headaches, excessive drowsiness, and/or seizures

Influenza

The flu is a highly contagious viral illness that tends to occur in epidemics during the winter. It is spread by the coughs and sneezes of infected people and also by direct contact with contaminated articles such as handkerchiefs. About 24–48 hours after exposure to the infection, you develop a sudden fever, shivering, headache, dry cough, muscle aches, exhaustion, and sore eyes and throat. Although you will begin to feel better after 4–5 days, you may feel tired and continue coughing for several weeks.

 ## See your doctor first

Arrange to see your doctor if:

- You are frail or elderly, have heart or lung problems, or have another chronic illness such as diabetes

What you can do yourself

Although you can't shorten a bout of the flu, these measures will help relieve the worst symptoms.

- Rest for a few days and avoid any unnecessary activity. As you begin to feel better, gradually increase what you do.

- Drink plenty of fluids, such as water or fruit juice. If you don't feel like eating, have nourishing fluids such as chicken soup and broths.

- Take an analgesic or flu remedy to relieve aches and pains (*see* DRUG REMEDIES, right).

- To relieve the "stuffed-up" feeling, use a steam inhalation (*see* PRACTICAL TECHNIQUE, p.79).

- Warm or chilled drinks soothe a sore throat. Try making a warm honey and lemon drink (*see* NATURAL REMEDIES, right).

- Don't smoke or allow anyone to smoke near you.

 ## Seek further medical advice

Arrange to see your doctor if:

- Your symptoms have not begun to clear up within a week
- You develop other symptoms, such as breathing problems, or cough up green, yellow, or bloody mucus

DRUG REMEDIES

Analgesics will reduce fever and help relieve headache and muscle aches. Take acetaminophen (*see* p.177) or ibuprofen (*see* p.185).

Cold and flu remedies (*see* p.180) contain drugs for various symptoms. They usually include an analgesic, such as acetaminophen, and a decongestant, to help you breathe more easily. Check the ingredients carefully. You should not use other remedies containing analgesics at the same time because of the risk of overdose.

NATURAL REMEDIES

Honey and lemon is a soothing drink for a sore throat. Use freshly squeezed lemon juice, liquid honey, and hot water.

Making the drink
Add a teaspoon each of honey and lemon juice to a cup of hot water.

PREVENTION

Immunization against flu is recommended for older people and those with low immunity and/or chronic health problems. A flu shot is usually given annually in the fall. Ask your doctor for advice.

Pertussis

Pertussis (whooping cough) is a severe bacterial infection that was common in children before immunization. Your child may be feverish and have cold symptoms 7–21 days after contact. Then spasms of coughing develop with a typical high-pitched "whoop" as the child breathes in. Coughing is usually worse at night and may trigger vomiting. The illness can be serious in small babies.

 See also Coughing, p.102; Croup, p.138.

WARNING

Seek immediate medical help if:
- Your child becomes drowsy, has seizures, or is choking
- Your child has breathing problems, or his or her lips or tongue turn blue during a coughing spasm

See your doctor first

Arrange to see your doctor immediately if you suspect that your child has pertussis.

What you can do yourself

Pertussis can be distressing, so follow these steps to make your child more comfortable.

- Be calm and reassuring. If your child is having trouble sleeping, try to share the care at night.

- Offer plenty of clear fluids. Try honey and lemon (*see* NATURAL REMEDIES, opposite page), but don't give honey to babies under 1 year.

- Give your child an analgesic (*see* DRUG REMEDIES, right) to reduce fever and discomfort. Don't use cough medicines – they will not help.

- Humidifying the room (*see* PRACTICAL TECHNIQUE, right) may help ease the cough.

- Offering your child soft, easy-to-swallow food in small portions will help prevent vomiting.

- Keep your home free of irritants such as tobacco smoke and aerosol sprays.

Seek further medical advice

Arrange to see your doctor:
- If your child's condition deteriorates
- To check that your child is fit to return to school; he or she may have coughing fits for several months after the illness

DRUG REMEDIES

Analgesics will help reduce discomfort and bring down a fever. Give acetaminophen (*see* p.177), available as liquid medicine or chewable pills, or ibuprofen (*see* p.185), available as liquid medicine. Make sure you ask your pharmacist to recommend an appropriate product for your child.

Acetaminophen
You can give medicine containing acetaminophen to a child over 2 years old.

PRACTICAL TECHNIQUE

Humidifying air in a room will soothe your child's air passages and help loosen mucus. Use one of the following methods.

- Place a humidifier by the child's bed, or hang a wet towel close to a radiator.
- Sit with your child in the bathroom and run hot water in the bath or shower to create steam.

PREVENTION

An effective vaccine that protects against pertussis is included in the childhood immunization series. Make sure your child is immunized according to the recommended schedule.

Chicken pox

Chicken pox is a highly infectious viral illness, most common in children, that causes an intensely itchy rash of blisters. Your child may generally feel unwell, with a headache and mild fever, just before the rash develops and for the first few days afterward. The first symptoms appear 1–3 weeks after contact with the infection, and most children are completely recovered 7–10 days later.

Chicken pox rash on a child

 ## See your doctor first

Arrange to see your doctor to confirm that your child has chicken pox.

What you can do yourself

Use these home treatments to make your child more comfortable and help prevent scratching, which can cause scars.

- If your child has a fever, take steps to reduce it (*see* FEVER IN CHILDREN, p.135). Offer your child plenty to drink throughout the day.

- Soothe itching by giving your child lukewarm baths twice a day. Try adding baking soda (sodium bicarbonate) or an oatmeal lotion to the bath water (*see* NATURAL REMEDIES, right).

- An antihistamine will reduce itching and help your child sleep at night. You can also soothe his or her skin with calamine lotion (*see* DRUG REMEDIES, right).

- Cut your child's nails short to reduce damage from scratching. Give him or her cotton gloves to wear at night to prevent scratching during sleep.

- To soothe spots in your child's mouth, get him or her to rinse with half a teaspoon of salt in a cup of warm water, being careful that he or she does not swallow the solution. Encourage your child to keep brushing his or her teeth as normal.

- Your child will be more comfortable in light, loose, nonitchy clothing. Avoid wool.

- Keep your child away from school, and away from any woman who may be pregnant, for 5 days from the time when the blisters first appear.

 ### NATURAL REMEDIES

Baking soda (*see* p.179) reduces itching. Add 2 tablespoons to a bath one-third full.

Oatmeal products (*see* p.187) moisturize the skin; lotions can be used instead of soap.

 ### DRUG REMEDIES

Antihistamines (*see* p.178) will help to relieve the itching during and after a chicken pox infection. Apply liberally to the affected areas. You could try using a liquid sedative brand if itching makes sleep difficult for your child.

Calamine lotion (*see* p.179) is cooling and soothing, and also helps dry up blisters, aiding healing. Use it as needed.

Applying calamine
Use cotton balls and count the spots with your child as you dab on the lotion.

 ## Seek further medical advice

Arrange to see your doctor again if your child develops:

- Pus-filled spots and/or blisters near the eyes
- Earache or headache, breathing problems, drowsiness, or convulsions

Shingles

Shingles is caused by reactivation of the chicken pox virus, which lies dormant in anyone who has had chicken pox. It begins with pain or tingling in an area of skin on one side of your body or face, followed by a rash of small, fluid-filled blisters. You may also have a headache and fever. The blisters scab over and heal within a few weeks, but the area may be painful for months afterward. Shingles is more common in later life. Stress, ill health, or sunlight can trigger an attack, but you can't catch shingles from contact with chicken pox.

Shingles rash

 ## See your doctor first

Arrange to see your doctor to confirm that you have shingles. See your doctor urgently if shingles has developed close to an eye.

What you can do yourself

Use these home treatments to make yourself feel better while you get over an attack of shingles.

- Rest as much as you can to speed your recovery.

- While you have a fever, drink plenty of fluids.

- Take an analgesic to relieve pain, headache, and fever (*see* DRUG REMEDIES, right). A cold compress (a cloth soaked in ice-cold water) may help relieve pain and tingling in your skin.

- If you have blisters on your body, take lukewarm baths 2–3 times a day. Add baking soda (sodium bicarbonate) or use an oatmeal product (*see* NATURAL REMEDIES, right) to soothe your skin. Wash any blisters on your face gently with soap and water.

- Until all the blisters are dry, avoid skin-to-skin contact with anyone who has not had chicken pox, because they could catch the virus from you.

 ## Seek further medical advice

Arrange to see your doctor again if:

- Your blisters become pus-filled and spread
- You develop severe headaches or vomiting
- Analgesics do not control the pain, or pain persists after the blisters have cleared

DRUG REMEDIES

Analgesics will relieve fever as well as pain. Use acetaminophen (*see* p.177), aspirin (*see* p.179), or ibuprofen (*see* p.185). Ask your pharmacist for advice on which product to use.

NATURAL REMEDIES

Baking soda (*see* p.179) can also help reduce itching. Add 4 tablespoons (about one cup) to a bath two-thirds full.

Oatmeal products (*see* p.187) are soothing for itchy, blistered skin. Add oatmeal oil to your bath or use the lotion instead of soap.

PREVENTION

Preventing attacks If you are susceptible to shingles, try the following measures:

- If you are prone to stress (a trigger for an attack of shingles), try using deep breathing exercises and muscle relaxation techniques to help you relax (*see* PRACTICAL TECHNIQUES, pp.20–21).
- Be careful to protect your skin from strong sunlight (*see* PREVENTION: SAFETY IN THE SUN, p.47).

SKIN, HAIR, AND NAIL PROBLEMS

Impetigo

Impetigo is a common skin infection that mainly affects children. It can appear anywhere on the body but most often develops on the face, especially around the nose and mouth. Red, weepy sores develop; the sores then blister and burst, and dry out to form an itchy, honey-colored crust. Caused by bacterial infection, impetigo is highly contagious and is spread by touch. The bacteria are present in small numbers on healthy skin, but impetigo tends to develop when there are minor cuts or scrapes that allow the bacteria to get under the skin.

Impetigo sores

 ## See your doctor first

Make an appointment to see your doctor to confirm impetigo. The doctor will probably prescribe antibiotics.

What you can do yourself

Impetigo usually clears up promptly with antibiotic treatment, but the following measures will speed recovery and reduce the risk of the sores spreading.

 ● Wash the affected area carefully (*see* PRACTICAL TECHNIQUE, right).

● Make sure your child has towels and washcloths for his or her own use. Change them daily and wash them in very hot water. Encourage your child to wash his or her hands frequently, drying them properly each time.

● Remind your child not to touch or pick the scabs or suck his or her fingers. Trim his or her nails to help prevent scratching.

● If your doctor prescribes an antibiotic drug or cream, make sure you give your child the complete course. Do not stop as soon as the impetigo appears to be better.

● Keep your child away from other children until there is no longer any crusting over the sores. Your child can then return to school or day care.

PRACTICAL TECHNIQUE

Washing infected areas Use the following procedure to soften and remove crusts and help the skin heal. (If you are using an antibiotic ointment, do this before you apply the ointment.)

● Soak the affected area by applying a clean washcloth soaked in warm water. Hold it over the skin for 1–2 minutes, being careful not to rub the rash. Pat the skin dry with a towel. Repeat this several times a day, washing your hands afterward.
● Do not cover the blisters. They will heal better if you leave them exposed to the air.

 ## Seek further medical advice

Arrange to see your doctor again if:

● The sores spread or enlarge
● The impetigo rash has not begun to clear within a few days
● Your child develops a fever or starts to pass red- or brown-colored urine

Scabies

Scabies is an infestation caused by a mite that burrows just under the skin surface. At first you will have intense itching, which is worse at night. You may then notice little bumps and tiny, pencil-like lines (burrows); these usually develop between the fingers and toes and on the elbows and wrists, but may occur anywhere on your skin. Scabies is troublesome rather than serious. Anyone can catch it, regardless of age and personal hygiene, through any type of skin-to-skin contact or simply by sharing bedding, towels, or clothing.

Scabies infestation on a hand and fingers

See your doctor first

Make an appointment to see your doctor if you think that you have scabies. He or she will check if you have the condition and prescribe the appropriate medication.

What you can do yourself

For best results, start scabies treatment as soon as the symptoms appear. This may be anything up to 8 weeks after infestation, and the itching can last for several weeks.

 • Use a prescription cream or lotion for treating scabies (see DRUG REMEDIES, right).

 • You can relieve itching with calamine lotion and/or take an antihistamine if itching is making it difficult for you to sleep (see DRUG REMEDIES, right).

• Make sure other people in the home and close friends are treated, even if they are not showing signs of scabies. Ask your physician to provide enough treatment for all household members.

• Scabies mites can live for 1–2 days in clothes and bedding. To kill the mites, wash clothes, bed linen, and towels in hot water and dry in a tumble dryer if possible. Wash personal items such as hairbrushes as well.

• Vacuum carpets, rugs, furniture, and cushions because they may harbor the scabies mites. Use a disposable bag in your vacuum cleaner and discard the bag afterward. If you have a bagless vacuum cleaner, empty it and wash it out after use.

DRUG REMEDIES

Scabies lotions usually contain the antiparasitic drugs lindane or permethrin. Your doctor will prescribe an appropriate preparation. Usually, the treatment is applied to your entire body (but not your head and face). Trim your nails short and apply it under your nail tips. Babies under 2 years and elderly people may need their face and scalp to be treated as well. The preparation is usually left on overnight and then washed off in the morning. A second application may be necessary, depending on the type of lotion used and your symptoms.

Antihistamines (see p.178) can help relieve itching. Sedative types make you drowsy, and are particularly useful at night.

Calamine lotion (see p.179) helps relieve the itchiness that occurs in scabies.

Relieving itching
Itching can persist for several weeks after the infestation has cleared up, so you may need to continue using calamine and/or an antihistamine.

Seek further medical advice

Arrange to see your doctor if:

• You are still itching more than 2 weeks after finishing your course of treatment
• The rash becomes sore and starts to ooze

Urticaria

Urticaria, or hives, is an intensely itchy rash of white or yellow swellings (wheals) surrounded by red, inflamed skin. It is usually caused by an allergic reaction, which can be triggered by a range of factors, such as certain foods or medicines, insect bites, or stings. People with hay fever or asthma are more susceptible. Hives can also be caused by stress, or have no obvious cause.

 See also **Anaphylactic shock**, p.159.

WARNING

Seek immediate medical help if you have urticaria and:

● You become breathless or hoarse, or start to wheeze
● Your lips or tongue swell and/or you have difficulty swallowing

 ## See your doctor first

Make an appointment to see your doctor to confirm that you have urticaria and/or to check whether you are taking medication that could be triggering the attack.

What you can do yourself

Urticaria is extremely uncomfortable, but the following measures will help relieve irritation and soothe the skin. Attacks are usually short-lived, but some people have persistent symptoms.

● Take an antihistamine to reduce itching and swelling (*see* DRUG REMEDIES, right).

● Take a cool shower to reduce the redness and "heat" of the rash. Alternatively, hold a cool compress (a clean washcloth soaked in cool water and wrung out) against the rash for a few minutes at a time. Keep reapplying for about 30 minutes.

● You can also relieve itching with calamine lotion (*see* DRUG REMEDIES, right).

● Try an oatmeal bath oil (*see* NATURAL REMEDIES, right) to relieve itchy skin.

● Minimize irritation by wearing loose-fitting, lightweight clothes made of natural fibers.

 ## Seek further medical advice

Arrange to see your doctor again if:

● Urticaria is not responding to treatment

DRUG REMEDIES

Antihistamines (*see* p.178) control allergic swelling and itching. You may need to try several types to find out which works best for you. The drug may need to be taken regularly for a prolonged attack of hives. Ask your pharmacist for advice.

Calamine lotion (*see* p.179) is a soothing preparation with a cooling effect. Using a cotton ball, dab it onto the rash 2–3 times a day.

NATURAL REMEDIES

Oatmeal products (*see* p.187) are often effective for soothing itchy skin. Add oatmeal oil to lukewarm bath water and soak for 10–20 minutes.

PREVENTION

Preventing urticaria If you have recurrent attacks, try these measures of prevention.

● Keep a diary of attacks, and try to identify any foods, medicines, or other factors that may trigger them. Once you find a trigger, you can try to avoid it.
● If you think stress is a contributory factor, try self-help techniques (*see* STRESS, pp.20–21).

Acne

Many teenagers have acne, and for some it is a distressing and persistent problem. Outbreaks of pimples, blackheads, whiteheads, and cysts occur on the face and sometimes on the chest and back. The cause is a surge of hormones during puberty that stimulates the oil-producing glands in the skin, making them prone to blockage and infection. Acne tends to clear up over time, but the pimples may leave scars. Attacks of acne in adults can be triggered by factors such as stress, changes in the weather, and using certain cosmetics.

What you can do yourself

There are various ways to tackle acne. Start treatment early to reduce the risk of scarring.

- Try a treatment containing benzoyl peroxide to reduce pimples (*see* DRUG REMEDIES, right).

- Gently wash affected areas twice a day with lukewarm water and a nonoily, perfume-free soap. Shampoo your hair daily and keep your hair off your face. Don't use hair products such as conditioners.

- Avoid covering affected areas with tight-fitting clothing, and do not wear hats.

- Don't squeeze pimples – they may get infected and spread. Be careful not to nick pimples when shaving.

- Avoid oil-based cosmetics and creams and opt for noncomedogenic products, which do not block pores. Go without makeup for 1 or 2 days a week.

- Try not to rub or touch your face absent-mindedly while you are absorbed in something such as watching TV or reading a book. Keep the phone away from your face when talking.

- Include plenty of healthy foods such as fruit and vegetables in your diet (*see* NATURAL REMEDIES, right).

- If stress makes your acne worse, try strategies that help reduce stress in your life (*see* pp.20–21).

 ### Seek medical advice

Arrange to see your doctor if:

- Your acne has not improved, or is spreading and is red and weepy, after you have used self-help remedies for 2 months
- You are a woman, and you also have hair growing on your face and are having irregular menstrual periods

DRUG REMEDIES

Benzoyl peroxide (*see* p.179), used every day, is an effective treatment for mild to moderate acne. It reduces inflammation, helps destroy bacteria, and prevents new pimples from forming. However, it may take up to 2 months before your skin responds to treatment. Use gel or lotion if you have oily skin; use cream for dry skin. Start with a low-strength type and go on to a higher strength if necessary. Continue the treatment until your acne clears up. Don't use benzoyl peroxide near your mouth or eyes.

Using benzoyl peroxide
Apply the treatment carefully, taking it slightly beyond the area of the pimples to prevent them from spreading.

NATURAL REMEDIES

Healthy foods are believed to support the immune system and maintain healthy skin. Boost your diet with lean meat, oily fish such as salmon, fruit, leafy and dark green vegetables, wheat germ, walnuts, sunflower seeds, and flaxseed.

Eczema

Eczema causes patches of dry, intensely itchy skin, which usually appear on the face, hands, wrists, and scalp, and in the creases of the knees and elbows. Repeated scratching may leave the skin cracked and open to infection. Eczema is often linked to allergies and asthma. It usually develops in infancy and disappears by the early teenage years, but adults may have relapses triggered by factors such as stress, dust mites, and some foods.

Eczema on the inside of an arm

 See also Stress, pp.20–21; Hay fever, p.80; Food intolerance, p.113.

 ## See your doctor first

Make an appointment to see your doctor even if you are fairly sure that you have eczema.

What you can do yourself

Although there is no cure for eczema, you can take these steps to help control the symptoms.

 ● Bathe only once a day using warm not hot water, and don't use perfumed bath products. Use a moisturizer instead of soap or add an oatmeal oil to the bath (*see* NATURAL REMEDIES, right). Afterward, apply moisturizer to soften and seal moisture into your skin. Reapply it generously throughout the day to the affected areas (*see* DRUG REMEDIES, right).

 ● Trim your nails or put on cotton gloves at night to prevent scratching. Try taking a sedative antihistamine to relieve itching and help you sleep (*see* DRUG REMEDIES, right).

● Wear cotton clothing next to your skin and avoid synthetic fabrics and wool. Wash clothes in non-allergenic laundry soaps, and rinse them well.

 ● For small, resistant patches of eczema, use a mild hydrocortisone cream to relieve inflammation (*see* DRUG REMEDIES, right).

 ## Seek further medical advice

Arrange to see your doctor again if:

● The eczema is not improving with treatment after a week, or is red, weepy, hot, or painful

DRUG REMEDIES

Moisturizers (*see* p.187) can be used instead of soap for washing. Rub water-based cream or ointment on your skin, rinse well, and pat yourself dry. Apply water-based cream liberally to patches of eczema throughout the day.

Antihistamines (*see* p.178), in liquid form for children and as pills for adults, relieve itching; the sedative brands will also help you sleep.

Hydrocortisone cream (*see* p.184) can be used for eczema but for no longer than a week. Apply sparingly, and not to your face unless your doctor tells you otherwise. Do not use the cream on children under 2 without medical advice.

PREVENTION

Avoiding triggers Certain factors can trigger eczema. Try to avoid any that affect you.

● Wear cotton-lined rubber or disposable gloves when using chemicals such as detergents and dyes.
● Follow practical advice on reducing allergens in your home (*see* PREVENTION, p.103).
● If you suspect that certain foods trigger eczema, try excluding them temporarily (*see* PRACTICAL TECHNIQUE: ELIMINATION DIET, p.113). Consult a doctor or nutritionist before eliminating foods from a child's diet.

Psoriasis

In psoriasis, patches of red, thickened skin with silvery scales develop, usually on the elbows, knees, scalp, and trunk. These areas can be itchy and painful. Your nails may become rough and pitted, and, less commonly, a form of arthritis develops. Psoriasis can be a persistent problem, and tends to run in families. Stress, infections such as a sore throat, and skin injuries may trigger an attack or make it worse.

Psoriasis on an elbow

See also **Disfigured or brittle nails**, p.53.

See your doctor first

Make an appointment to see your doctor if you think that you have psoriasis.

What you can do yourself

The following measures may be all you need to treat a mild case of psoriasis. Check with your doctor before using them with prescribed treatment.

- Take a daily bath in warm water to soak off the scales. Try using a coal tar preparation (*see* DRUG REMEDIES, right) to soften the scales.

- Apply a moisturizer to lubricate and soften scaly patches of skin (*see* DRUG REMEDIES, right).

- Don't scratch or rub patches of thickened skin. Using an oatmeal bath oil, or applying an aloe vera cream or gel, may help reduce itchiness (*see* NATURAL REMEDIES, right).

- Sunshine can help improve psoriasis but be careful not to burn. Sunburn can make it worse.

- If stress is making your psoriasis worse, try some deep breathing and muscle relaxation exercises (*see* PRACTICAL TECHNIQUES, pp.20–21).

Seek further medical advice

Arrange to see your doctor again if:

- Your psoriasis is not controlled by treatment
- Large areas of skin become red and inflamed, and you have a fever and feel unwell
- You develop joint pains

DRUG REMEDIES

Coal tar preparations (*see* p.180) help control psoriasis but have a strong smell. Add a coal tar solution to a daily bath; apply a cream 1–3 times a day; and use a coal tar shampoo. If you have thick scales on your scalp, use coal tar combined with salicylic acid to soften and remove them. If your skin becomes irritated, discontinue use. Coal tar makes skin more sensitive to ultraviolet light, so avoid exposing skin to sunlight after use.

Moisturizers (*see* p.187), such as water-based cream, should be rubbed gently into the skin as often as possible to relieve itching and loosen scales.

NATURAL REMEDIES

Oatmeal bath oils (*see* p.187) help soften scaly plaques and relieve itching.

Aloe vera creams and gels (*see* p.177) may help reduce dryness and itching in psoriasis. There is some evidence for their effectiveness but ask your doctor for advice before using them.

Using aloe vera
Apply aloe vera gel or cream thinly to irritated and itchy patches of skin and rub in lightly.

Rosacea

Rosacea is a flush or rash that comes and goes on your chin, nose, cheeks, and forehead. You may also have small bumps and pimples on your cheeks, sore eyes and eyelids, and, more rarely, a swollen, red nose. Rosacea is triggered by factors such as emotional stress, alcohol, or hot, spicy food. Flare-ups are due to inflammation of the tiny blood vessels under the skin but why rosacea develops in the first place is unknown. The problem seems to run in families; it mainly affects women aged 30–55, and can become permanent.

Rosacea rash on cheek

 ## See your doctor first

Make an appointment to see your doctor if you think you have rosacea.

What you can do yourself

Flare-ups are usually caused by something that makes you flush or overheat. There are several things you can do to reduce the symptoms.

- Put a cold compress (a washcloth soaked in ice-cold water) on the flushed areas to cool your skin.

 - Some foods and drinks trigger attacks. Try to identify which, if any, are affecting you (*see* PRACTICAL TECHNIQUE, right).

- Use mild cleansers and avoid any that contain alcohol. Don't rub your face hard or use a washcloth.

- Bathing or showering in lukewarm, rather than hot, water is less likely to irritate the skin.

- Wear cotton rather than wool and dress in layers so you can remove a layer if you begin to feel hot.

- To minimize redness, try a green-tinted foundation; choose one that is specially formulated for sensitive skin. Camouflage creams are also available but you may need a specialist's advice on selecting and applying them.

- Use a moisturizer to protect your skin against the drying effects of cold weather.

- If you are a man with rosacea, use an electric shaver rather than shaving cream.

 ### PRACTICAL TECHNIQUE

Identifying trigger substances
This should help you to avoid particular foods and drinks, such as coffee, alcohol, and spicy food, that can cause flare-ups of rosacea.

- Keep a journal of your symptoms and what you have eaten when they occur.
- Try eliminating any suspect foods or drinks for up to 6 weeks to see if there is an improvement.
- Reintroduce foods and drinks one at a time, noting which provoke an attack and need to be avoided.

 ### PREVENTION

Avoiding attacks If you are prone to flushes, following the advice given here may help reduce the frequency and severity of attacks.

- Sunlight can cause flare-ups, so stay in the shade on hot summer days and wear a hat. When you are in the sun, use a sunscreen; a titanium dioxide sunblock (*see* DRUG REMEDIES: SUNSCREENS AND SUNBLOCKS, p.47) is less likely to irritate your skin.
- Avoid rapid changes of temperature – for example, going straight from the cold outdoors into a hot room.
- If you tend to have flare-ups of rosacea when you are feeling under stress, try practicing deep breathing exercises and muscle relaxation techniques (*see* PRACTICAL TECHNIQUES, pp.20–21).

Dry skin

When your skin lacks moisture it tends to be itchy and flaky. It may look red, rough, and scaly and, in severe cases, become cracked and inflamed. You are most likely to develop dry skin on your lower legs, arms, and the backs of your hands because these areas produce less of the natural oils that seal moisture into the skin. Your skin also becomes drier as you get older and during menopause. You may develop sore, rough, chapped skin on your face in dry, cold weather, or if your face gets wet repeatedly and is not dried properly.

What you can do yourself

There are plenty of easy-to-use remedies that reduce the discomfort of dry, itchy skin and improve its appearance. Use the following measures.

- Take baths rather than showers (which tend to strip oils from the skin) no more than once a day in warm, rather than hot, water. Don't use perfumed or medicated bath products or soaps.

 • Use moisturizing cream or ointment instead of soap (*see* DRUG REMEDIES, right).

 • Alternatively, use a bath oil containing oatmeal (*see* NATURAL REMEDIES, right).

 • After your bath, apply a moisturizing cream (*see* DRUG REMEDIES, right). Reapply it frequently to exposed areas such as your hands and face, especially after washing or if you are outdoors for long periods in cold weather. Keep tubes of cream around the house and at work to use during the day.

PREVENTION

Preventing dryness If your skin tends to get dry or chapped, try the following measures.

- Don't overheat your home. In centrally heated rooms keep the air moist by fitting humidifying devices to radiators, or put bowls of water near them.
- Wear rubber gloves for household cleaning and gloves for gardening and other outdoor activities.
- Limit sunbathing. Use a sunscreen (*see* DRUG REMEDIES: SUNSCREENS AND SUNBLOCKS, p.47) when you are out in the sun. At high altitudes, use a sunscreen formulated for skiing.
- Rinse your laundry well and don't use fabric conditioners; they may irritate your skin.

DRUG REMEDIES

Moisturizers (*see* p.187) can be used instead of soaps for washing and to protect and soothe dry skin. Use a water-based cream or emulsifying ointment, rather than a perfumed product, in the bath and when you wash. Rinse the product off thoroughly. Pat your skin with a towel (rather than rubbing), preserving a thin layer of moisture. Then apply more water-based cream to seal the moisture in.

Water-based cream
Apply water-based cream liberally to your skin while it is still moist after a bath.

NATURAL REMEDIES

Oatmeal bath oil (*see* OATMEAL PRODUCTS, p.187) is soothing and moisturizing for dry, itchy skin. Add it to a warm bath and soak for 10–20 minutes.

 ## Seek medical advice

Arrange to see your doctor if:

- You still have dry, chapped skin after trying the measures described above
- Your skin becomes inflamed and bleeds

Corns and calluses

Prolonged pressure or friction on the feet or hands can cause patches of hard skin – corns or calluses – to form. Corns tend to develop over the toe joints or between toes, often as a result of badly fitting shoes. Calluses may occur on the soles of your feet, usually due to uneven pressure when walking, or on your hands if you do heavy manual work or play a musical instrument. Corns and calluses protect the soft skin beneath, so you may not need to remove them unless they are painful.

Corn on toe joint

See your doctor or podiatrist first

Make an appointment to see your doctor or a podiatrist if you have corns and calluses and you also have diabetes or suffer from poor circulation.

What you can do yourself

First find out what has caused the corn or callus, because it will be easier to treat once the source of friction has been removed. Take the following steps to relieve the problem.

 ● Use a foam wedge to relieve pressure on corns between the toes, and corn pads (small rings of sponge) to protect corns in other areas. Corn and blister bandages will help to cushion and soften the skin (*see* DRUG REMEDIES, right).

● Soak the corn or callus in warm, soapy water for 10 minutes each day, then use a pumice stone to gently rub away the hard skin.

 ● Never cut or shave corns yourself. Instead, you can apply salicylic acid to soften the thickened skin gradually (*see* DRUG REMEDIES, right).

Seek further medical advice

Arrange to see your doctor if:

● Your corn or callus does not disappear with self-help measures
● The skin is becoming painful, red, swollen, or weepy, or an ulcer develops

DRUG REMEDIES

Corn and blister bandages (*see* p.180) contain a substance that absorbs moisture released by the skin. This forms a gel that cushions the area and also softens the skin so that the corn or callus can be removed easily.

Salicylic acid gels, lotions, or ointments (*see* p.188) can be used to soften calluses and corns, making them easier to remove. Products containing salicylic acid may burn surrounding skin, so apply them with care and follow the instructions carefully. Alternatively, use corn pads, which apply salicylic acid directly to the corn.

Moisturizers (*see* p.187) soften the skin, so calluses are less likely to develop. Apply water-based cream or emulsifying ointment to the hands and feet after washing and during the day.

PREVENTION

Preventing corns and calluses
The following measures will help protect your hands and feet from friction and pressure.

● Wear comfortable shoes that fit properly. Avoid high heels and pointed shoes. Make sure worn-down soles and heels are repaired promptly.
 ● If your soles are prone to calluses, cushion them with corn and blister bandages (*see* DRUG REMEDIES, above) or padding inside your shoe.
 ● Use a moisturizer regularly to keep your skin soft (*see* DRUG REMEDIES, above).
● Wear padded gloves when using tools or machinery.
● If you play a stringed instrument, it may help to put adhesive bandages on your fingertips for protection.

Warts and plantar warts

Warts are small, round growths on the skin that have a rough, cauliflower-like appearance and, sometimes, tiny black spots in the center. They are caused by a virus and tend to be most common in children and young adults. Warts are most likely to develop on your hands or on the soles of your feet; those that occur on the feet are called plantar warts. Although warts do not usually hurt, plantar warts may be painful because walking puts pressure on them – it may feel like having a pebble in your shoe.

 ## See your doctor first

Make an appointment to see your doctor if:

- You are not entirely certain that a new growth on your skin is a wart
- You have warts on your face or around the anus or genitals: these need special treatment

What you can do yourself

Most warts disappear eventually, but it can take a long time – sometimes years. Prompt treatment may, however, help prevent them from spreading or hurting and can clear them up completely.

 - A wart remover containing salicylic acid is usually effective (*see* DRUG REMEDIES, right).

 - Follow a treatment regimen using a pumice stone and wart remover until your wart has disappeared (*see* PRACTICAL TECHNIQUE, right).

- A soft insole inside your shoe may help to reduce the discomfort of a plantar wart.

- Don't scratch or pick at your warts – this may make them spread. Nail biting may also spread the infection, so try not to do it (*see* NAIL BITING, p.54).

 ## Seek further medical advice

Arrange to see your doctor if:

- Your wart does not respond to treatment
- The wart changes in appearance, bleeds, or becomes red, hot, and painful

DRUG REMEDIES

Salicylic acid gels, lotions, or ointments (*see* p.188) soften warts so that they can then be removed easily. Products containing salicylic acid can burn healthy skin, however, so you need to use them with care. Make sure that you apply them only to the wart and not to the surrounding skin.

PRACTICAL TECHNIQUE

Treating a wart You can remove a wart gradually by soaking it, rubbing it with a pumice stone, and applying a wart remover. Instructions for use vary, but most can be used as follows.

1 *First soak the wart for a few minutes in warm water to soften it. Then use a pumice stone to rub the surface of the wart gently. This will help to remove dead skin.*

Rub away dead skin from the surface of the wart

2 *Isolate the wart with a corn pad, or shield the surrounding skin with petroleum jelly. Apply the wart remover, then cover the treated wart with an adhesive bandage.*

Keep wart remover away from surrounding skin

3 *Once a week, rub away the treated surface with the pumice stone. Treat the wart until it disappears. (This may take several weeks.)*

Athlete's foot and jock itch

These are common fungal infections. Athlete's foot affects the skin between the toes, making it cracked, sore, and itchy with peeling areas. It may spread to the soles and toenails. Jock itch is an itchy, scaly, red rash in the groin, more common in men. Both infections thrive in warm, sweaty conditions. You can catch them from contact with an infected person or sharing items such as towels and footwear.

Athlete's foot between the toes

 See also Ringworm, p.48; Disfigured or brittle nails, p.53.

What you can do yourself

Both infections are easy to treat yourself. Keep using the good hygiene practices outlined below to help prevent fungal infections recurring.

 Athlete's foot
● Treat the infection with an antifungal cream and/or powder (*see* DRUG REMEDIES, right).

● Wash your feet twice daily, making sure you dry thoroughly between your toes afterward. Use a separate towel just for drying your feet, and wash the towel frequently.

● Wear socks made from natural fibers and change them at least once a day. Women should avoid wearing pantyhose and tights, especially those that are restrictive around the feet.

● Wear well-ventilated shoes made from natural rather than synthetic materials; open-toed sandals are particularly good.

● Wear flip-flops when walking around communal changing areas, such as at swimming pools.

 Jock itch
● Apply an antifungal treatment to the infected area (*see* DRUG REMEDIES, right).

● Wash your groin regularly, drying it thoroughly but avoiding chafing. Use a separate towel to dry this area, and launder the towel frequently.

● Don't wear tight-fitting pants or underwear, or underwear made from synthetic fabrics. Cotton underpants or boxer shorts are best as these fabrics allow air to circulate. Change them daily.

DRUG REMEDIES

Antifungal drugs (*see* p.178), such as clotrimazole, miconazole, or terbinafine, are used to treat athlete's foot and jock itch. They are available as a cream or a fine powder spray (which is usually easier to apply). Most are applied twice daily. The infection should start to clear up within a week, although it may take several weeks longer to disappear completely. To help treat athlete's foot, you can also dust inside your shoes and socks with an antifungal foot powder.

Powder spray
Apply the powder after washing and drying your feet carefully. Spray generously, paying particular attention to areas between the toes.

 ## Seek medical advice

Arrange to see your doctor if:

● The affected area becomes hot and red, or starts weeping
● The infection does not clear up after you have tried self-help treatment

Boils

A boil begins as a small, red, painful lump under the skin, which swells as pus builds up inside. The area is usually warm to the touch and throbs. The cause is most commonly an infection in a hair follicle or oil gland in the skin; the buttocks, thighs, armpits, face, and neck are particularly susceptible. Most boils come to a head and burst, releasing pus, after which the skin heals. Some boils, however, gradually subside without bursting. Sometimes, a cluster of connected boils forms; this is known as a carbuncle.

 ## See your doctor first

Make an appointment to see your doctor if:

- You think you have a carbuncle
- You have diabetes

What you can do yourself

There are several simple measures that you can take to reduce discomfort and speed up healing.

- Take an analgesic such as acetaminophen if the boil is painful (*see* DRUG REMEDIES, right).

- Wash the area thoroughly every day. Dry it well.

- Help bring the boil to a head by applying a warm compress several times a day (*see* PRACTICAL TECHNIQUE, right).

- Don't squeeze the boil or try to burst it with a needle because this may spread the infection; let it burst or subside by itself.

- If the boil has burst, cover the area with a gauze dressing. Wash the area thoroughly and change the dressing regularly until the skin has healed.

- Keep your own towels and washcloths separate to avoid spreading the infection to other people.

- Bedding or clothing that comes into contact with the boil should be washed in very hot, preferably boiling, water.

- Wash your hands thoroughly before handling food, and make sure the boil is covered with an adhesive bandage or other dressing. The bacteria that cause boils can also cause food poisoning.

- Avoid contact sports until the boil has gone.

DRUG REMEDIES

Analgesics, such as acetaminophen (*see* p.177), can relieve the pain of an inflamed or irritating boil.

PRACTICAL TECHNIQUE

Applying a warm compress
Use this treatment up to 4 times a day to help bring the boil to a head and encourage it to burst.

- Soak a clean cloth in a bowl of warm water, then wring it out and place it over the boil. Soaking the compress repeatedly to rewarm it, continue to reapply it for about 30 minutes.
- Cover the boil with a gauze dressing.
- Keep using the compress for a few days after the boil has burst, to encourage it to drain.

Applying heat
Heat a cloth in warm water and hold it over the boil until it cools.

 ## Seek further medical advice

Arrange to see your doctor if:

- The boil has not begun to disappear after a week of using self-help measures
- It becomes very painful and/or enlarges
- You are getting recurrent boils
- You develop a fever and feel generally ill

Heat rash and sunburn

Heat rash, also known as prickly heat, is an itchy, red, pimply rash that may develop around your neck and on your chest, back, armpits, and groin in hot or humid weather, particularly during exercise. Babies who overheat because they are dressed too warmly, or because of a fever, are particularly susceptible to heat rash. Sunburn is the result of overexposure to sunshine or to ultraviolet rays on a tanning bed. If you are mildly burned you will have red, sore skin on areas such as your shoulders, arms, thighs, back, and nose, which may begin to itch and peel a few days later. More severe sunburn can cause blistering and pain. Although you are most likely to burn in hot summer sun, you can also burn on an overcast day, in water, or at high altitudes. Babies, children, and fair-skinned people with red or blond hair and blue eyes are most at risk.

 See also Fever (children), p.135; Fever (babies), p.142.

 ## See your doctor first

Arrange to see a doctor immediately if:

- You are not sure that a baby has heat rash, or a baby has a rash with fever
- You have severe sunburn with extensive blistering, and/or feel unwell, with vomiting, fever, confusion, or headaches
- A child or baby gets sunburned

What you can do yourself

You can treat an attack of heat rash or a case of mild sunburn with the following measures. They will make your skin feel more comfortable and help speed your recovery.

Heat rash
- Loosen or remove your clothing and find a cool place to sit, such as an air-conditioned room. If available, use a fan to help cool yourself down, and avoid any activity that might make you sweat.
- Have plenty of cool, nonalcoholic drinks.
- Apply a cold compress to affected areas. Soak a sponge or washcloth in cold water, wring it out, and apply to your skin. Use it as often as needed.

 - If your baby develops heat rash, take immediate steps to cool him or her down (*see* PRACTICAL TECHNIQUE, right).

- To soothe dry, itchy skin, try taking frequent, lukewarm baths with oatmeal bath oil (*see* p.187). Pat your skin dry afterward.

 PRACTICAL TECHNIQUE

Treating a baby with heat rash
A baby with heat rash needs to be cooled down promptly. The rash should then disappear.

- Take off your baby's clothes and diaper and lay him or her on a cotton sheet or towel to let the air circulate around the skin. Allow your baby to kick freely until he or she cools down.
- Don't use ointments, lotions, or powders because they may block the pores and aggravate the rash.
- If your baby has a fever, give him or her plenty of fluids and take steps to reduce body temperature (*see* FEVER [BABIES], p.142).

Cooling down
Once your baby is undressed, the air will help cool his or her skin.

 NATURAL REMEDIES

Aloe vera (*see* p.177) is found in many after-sun lotions and is also available as a gel. It has soothing properties that help cool sunburned skin and relieve dryness and irritation. However, don't use gels or cream to treat heat rash.

What you can do yourself *continued...*

- While you have a heat rash, don't use antiperspirants, perfumes, lotions, or creams, which may irritate your skin or block your pores.

- When the weather is warm, wear lightweight, loose clothes made of natural fibers such as cotton.

- If you are prone to heat rash, acclimatize yourself gradually whenever you move from a cool climate to a hot one. Increase the time you spend in the heat over several days.

- To prevent heat rash in a baby, avoid overdressing or using too many blankets. (Check by feeling the back of your baby's neck — it should be warm but not sweaty.) On hot days, keep your baby in cool, shady areas and give him or her plenty to drink.

Sunburn

- Stay out of the sun while you have a sunburn. If you do go outdoors, wear cool, lightweight clothes that cover the burns completely.

- Don't pick at peeling skin; let any blisters burst on their own.

- Have a cool bath and add about 4 tablespoons of baking soda (*see* p.179) to the bath water. Pat yourself dry with a soft towel.

- You may find a cold compress soothing. Soak a soft cloth in cold water, wring it out, and apply it gently to your sunburned skin. Repeat as often as necessary throughout the day.

- Calamine lotion may help to cool sunburned skin (*see* DRUG REMEDIES, right).

- Try an aloe vera lotion or gel to soothe your skin (*see* NATURAL REMEDIES, opposite page). Wait until the skin has been cooled down before applying moisturizers, which hold in the heat of the burn.

✚ Seek further medical advice

Arrange to see your doctor if:

- A heat rash does not fade within 2–3 days
- A baby is still feverish after you have used cooling methods

DRUG REMEDIES

Calamine lotion (*see* p.179) has a cooling effect on sore, itchy sunburned skin. Dab it on with cotton balls as often as needed.

Sunscreens and sunblocks (*see* p.189) have different sun protection factors (SPFs) for different skin types — the fairer your skin, the higher the factor. Most people need an SPF of 15 or higher. (Much higher factors may be needed at high altitudes, when skiing, for example.) Use a sunscreen even in the shade and on cloudy days. Apply sunscreen 30 minutes before you go outside and reapply frequently, especially after swimming. Use a total sunblock with zinc oxide or titanium dioxide if you have very fair skin and for all children. Don't use sunscreens or sunblocks on a baby under 6 months.

PREVENTION

Safety in the sun The effects of the sun on your skin don't always show straight away, so you may not realize you are burning. The following measures will help protect you from sunburn.

- Whenever your skin is exposed to the sun, use sunscreen or sunblock (*see* DRUG REMEDIES, above).
- Don't go out in summer sunshine when it is at its strongest, between 11am and 3pm.
- Don't use tanning beds.
- Be especially careful when you are close to water or snow because the reflected sunlight increases the likelihood of getting sunburned.
- Keep babies out of the sun completely. Use a sunshade or sit them in the shade.
- Wear loose, lightweight pants and tops with sleeves, and also a hat, if you are out in the sun for long periods. Some clothes are now labeled with an ultraviolet protection factor (UPF), indicating their effectiveness at blocking the sun's rays.

Sun protection
Choose a hat that shades your child's face and neck and apply sunscreen to skin exposed to the sun.

Ringworm

Ringworm produces round, red, itchy, scaly patches on your skin that enlarge over a week or so to form raised red rings. It can occur anywhere, but if it affects the scalp, it also causes broken hair and hair loss. Ringworm isn't caused by a worm – it is a fungal infection caught by direct contact with an infected person or pet, or from contaminated items such as towels and hairbrushes.

Patch of ringworm on the skin

 See also Athlete's foot and jock itch, p.44; Disfigured or brittle nails, p.53.

 ## See your doctor first

Make an appointment to see your doctor if:

● You have many patches of ringworm or you have ringworm of the scalp

What you can do yourself

You may be able to clear up ringworm yourself using the following measures. Otherwise, use them with treatment that your doctor prescribes.

 ● If you have only a small area of ringworm, try an antifungal cream (*see* DRUG REMEDIES, right). Wash your hands thoroughly after touching the patches.

 ● Keep your skin clean and dry and try not to scratch. An oatmeal bath oil may help soothe itching (*see* NATURAL REMEDIES, right).

● To prevent the infection from spreading to others or reinfecting yourself, wash clothes, bedding, and towels that you have worn or used recently. If you have scalp ringworm, also wash brushes, combs, and hats after each use.

● Don't touch animals that show signs of infection, such as hair loss. If you suspect your pet has ringworm, make sure it has veterinary treatment.

● If you have scalp ringworm, use a mild shampoo such as baby shampoo, and wash and dry your hair gently without using a hair dryer. Don't use gels, mousses, or other hair products on your hair.

● You don't need to stay away from other people but avoid contact sports until you have had at least 4 days of antifungal treatment.

 ### DRUG REMEDIES

Antifungal creams (*see* ANTIFUNGAL DRUGS, p.178) can be used to treat small areas of ringworm if you are not already using a drug or cream prescribed by your doctor. Apply the cream as directed on the package. The infection should begin to clear up within a week or two, although it may take several more weeks to completely disappear. Continue using the cream for several days after your skin has started to look healthy again.

 ### NATURAL REMEDIES

Oatmeal bath oils (*see* OATMEAL PRODUCTS, p.187) can help to relieve itching. Relax in the bath for 10–20 minutes. Make sure you dry yourself thoroughly afterward, because fungal infections thrive on warm, damp skin.

 ## Seek further medical advice

Arrange to see your doctor if:

● The patches have not started responding to treatment within a week
● Your skin is red and the patches are oozing and sore
● You have a large swelling on your scalp that is oozing pus and shedding hair

Dandruff

In this harmless but sometimes embarrassing condition, excessive amounts of skin cells flake off the scalp. They show up as white flakes in your hair, and on your shoulders if you wear dark clothes. Your scalp may also be itchy and red, and your eyelids, nose, and forehead may be affected. Dandruff is usually associated with the growth of a yeastlike fungus on the scalp, or it can be a mild form of seborrheic dermatitis – a scaly, itchy rash that can also affect the eyelids. Dandruff is more common in men and may be made worse by stress, illness, and some hair products. Scaly, flaking skin on a baby's scalp is known as cradle cap.

 See also **Itchy eyes**, p.56; **Cradle cap**, p.151.

What you can do yourself

Dandruff can usually be controlled with the treatments below. You may need to repeat them occasionally, because the condition tends to recur.

- Use an antidandruff shampoo (*see* DRUG REMEDIES, right) and wash your hair in warm rather than hot water. Massage the shampoo into your scalp and make sure you leave it on long enough to work – generally about 3–5 minutes. Rinse thoroughly afterward.

- Keep using the brand of antidandruff shampoo that you find works for you. If you develop itchiness or a rash, however, stop using the shampoo immediately and try switching to one with a different active ingredient.

- Don't blow-dry your hair because it may aggravate the dandruff.

- Avoid alcohol-based hair products such as hair sprays, which tend to dry out the scalp, and mousses, gels, and dyes, which may increase irritation and make dandruff worse.

- Treat itchy, flaky skin on your eyelids (blepharitis) with a special cleaning regime (*see* PRACTICAL TECHNIQUE: CLEANING YOUR EYELIDS, p.56).

DRUG REMEDIES

Antidandruff shampoos (*see* p.177) should clear up your dandruff within a few weeks. Follow the instructions carefully because different brands have different treatment advice. Shampoos may contain pyrithione zinc, selenium sulfide, or ketoconazole, which is particularly effective. Alternatively, use a shampoo that contains coal tar, or sulfur and salicylic acid.

Shampooing
After shampooing, rinse your hair thoroughly to remove every trace of antidandruff shampoo.

 ## Seek medical advice

Arrange to see your doctor if:

- The dandruff does not clear up after you have been using these home treatments
- You develop sensitivity to an antidandruff shampoo that persists for more than a few days
- Your scalp becomes red and develops sore patches or crusts

Head lice

Head lice are gray-brown insects about the size of a sesame seed that live on or close to the scalp. They lay eggs that hatch into more lice, and the oval off-white egg cases (nits) remain glued to the bases of hairs. They look like dandruff but can't be brushed off. Because head lice are easily passed on by close contact they can affect anyone, but are more common in children. You may see your child scratching his or her head, although itching may not develop until some time after infection.

Nits in hair

 ## See your doctor first

Make an appointment to see your doctor if you aren't sure whether you have lice, or if you have lice but don't know which treatment to use.

What you can do yourself

You can treat head lice yourself, but you only need to do so if you find live lice in the hair.

- To detect head lice, use detection combing (*see* PRACTICAL TECHNIQUE, right). If you find lice, check family members and tell anyone who has had recent close contact with you or your child so they can be treated if necessary.

- Apply a head lice preparation to kill the lice (*see* DRUG REMEDIES, right).

- If you are pregnant or breast-feeding, or treating a baby under 6 months old, you should not use head lice preparations. Instead, you can use repeated detection combing (*see* PRACTICAL TECHNIQUE, right), which is also an option if you prefer not to use insecticides.

- Head lice die quickly once they leave the scalp but, as a precaution, wash brushes, combs, towels, and pillowcases, and don't share hats, scarves, brushes, and combs with anyone else.

 ## Seek further medical advice

Arrange to see your doctor if:

- You find live lice 2 or 3 days after the second application of a head lice preparation or after combing regularly for 2 weeks

PRACTICAL TECHNIQUE

Detection combing It is difficult to find lice by just looking in the hair, so use the following process. It takes about 15–30 minutes.

- Shampoo and rinse your hair and apply a generous amount of conditioner. Comb with an ordinary comb.
- Insert a detection comb at the hair roots, with the teeth flat against the scalp. Draw it up to the hair tips.
- Check the comb after each stroke, and remove any lice by wiping it on a tissue.
- Make sure you cover the entire head, combing over a white towel so you can see any lice that fall.
- If you find lice, rinse your hair, let it dry, and apply a head lice preparation. Alternatively, rinse and repeat combing. Repeat 3 more times at 4-day intervals. If you find live lice in a subsequent session, repeat combing 3 more times, at 4-day intervals, until none are seen.

Combing method
Work backward and forward and from side to side over the whole head.

DRUG REMEDIES

Head lice preparations (*see* p.184) kill lice. Normally, you rub the preparation into the hair and scalp and leave it on for a set period of time, depending on the particular product. You then shampoo your hair and comb out the dead lice. A second treatment may be necessary.

Unwanted or ingrown hair

Excessive hair growth (hirsutism) can affect both sexes, but is usually only a problem for women. Some women are naturally more hairy than others and may have unwanted hair on their face, and hair growing thickly on their arms, pubic area, abdomen, and thighs. Excessive hair growth can also occur during pregnancy and after menopause. More rarely, it is due to an underlying illness or a drug. Ingrown hairs are often caused by hair-removal methods; as the hair grows again, it curls back into the skin, causing inflammation.

 ## See your doctor first

Make an appointment to see your doctor if:

- You have noticed a recent increase in facial or body hair, and/or you have other symptoms such as irregular or absent periods, deepening of the voice, and weight increase
- You think that the hair growth may be due to a prescribed medication

What you can do yourself

If you are concerned about excess hair, try the following cosmetic measures.

- Use a hair-bleaching cream to lighten hair on your face (see DRUG REMEDIES, right).

- Pluck with tweezers to remove stray hairs under your nose and on your chin.

- Shaving is better for larger areas such as the legs. You can use an electric shaver or wet razor, which gives a closer shave. You will need to shave daily to avoid stubble. Shaving does not cause hair to grow back more thickly. Alternatively, use a hair removal product (see DRUG REMEDIES, right).

- Waxing or sugaring is effective (see PRACTICAL TECHNIQUE, right) because hairs are pulled out at the root, and take up to 4 weeks to grow back. However, if you find waxing difficult, consult a beauty therapist.

- Ingrown hairs usually dislodge themselves if you let them grow out. If not, try to lift out the end of the hair with a needle that has been sterilized under a flame, or dissolve the hair with a hair removal product (see DRUG REMEDIES, right). Don't shave until any inflammation has gone.

 ### DRUG REMEDIES

Hair bleaches (see p.183) lighten facial hair and make it less noticeable against fair skin, but they are not as suitable for darker skins.

Hair-removal products (see p.184) include fast-acting creams and mousses that dissolve hair roots. Waxes and sugars pull out hair. Test products on a small area first in case of a reaction.

 ### PRACTICAL TECHNIQUE

Waxing Before waxing or sugaring, hairs need to be at least ¼in (5 mm) long and your skin clean, dry, and free of creams and oils. Be careful if you have to heat the wax; very hot wax can burn the skin.

1 *Apply a thin layer of wax or sugar paste on a small section of the area to be treated, in the direction of hair growth.*

2 *Place a fabric strip over the area and smooth it down. Holding the skin taut, pull off the strip against the direction of hair growth in one swift movement.*

3 *Continue until all the unwanted hair is removed, going back over areas of stubborn hairs. Apply an unperfumed moisturizing cream afterward. Avoid bathing or swimming until any redness has disappeared.*

Hair thinning and hair loss

Temporary hair loss often occurs after an illness or period of stress, or because of a skin infection such as ringworm. Chemical hair treatments, and hairstyles and hats that pull on the hair, can contribute to the problem. Some drugs and long-term illnesses cause hair loss, and women may lose hair temporarily after childbirth. Permanent hair loss is usually hereditary and can begin to affect men as early as in their twenties. Women who inherit the trait develop thin hair later in life but do not usually become bald.

 See also **Ringworm**, p.48.

 ## See your doctor first

Make an appointment to see your doctor if:

- You have been losing hair rapidly or in patches in recent weeks
- You think your hair loss may be due to a medication or an illness
- You are pulling your hair out

What you can do yourself

There is little you can do to prevent hereditary hair loss, but treatments may reverse some of its effects. For temporary hair loss, try the following to slow hair thinning and encourage regrowth.

- Fad diets and crash diets may contribute to hair loss. Make sure you include plenty of protein and iron in your diet (*see* NATURAL REMEDIES, right).

- Avoid using hair dyes and treatments to perm or straighten your hair. They contain chemicals that may make hair brittle and liable to break at the roots.

- Don't wear your hair in a style that pulls on your scalp, or wear a cap or hat continuously unless you have to wear headgear for your work.

- Let your hair dry naturally if possible, rather than using a hair dryer. Don't pull on your hair with a brush or comb when it is wet.

- If your hair is thinning, a good haircut can make a difference. Short, blunt cuts can make hair appear thicker. Some men prefer to cut their hair very short, or shave it off, to disguise a receding hairline.

- If you are in the early stages of hereditary hair loss, you can try a preparation containing minoxidil that may restore hair (*see* DRUG REMEDIES, right).

 ### NATURAL REMEDIES

Protein and iron Protein is essential for building and repairing tissues in the body, including hair. Make sure about one sixth of your total calorie intake is made up of foods such as meat, fish, cheese, and nuts. Iron also helps maintain healthy hair, so eat plenty of iron-rich foods such as grains, beans, fish, poultry, meat, and leafy green vegetables.

DRUG REMEDIES

Minoxidil preparations (*see* p.186) can slow down or prevent hereditary hair loss in a proportion of men and women. The treatment is applied twice daily and needs to be used continually, since its effect starts to wear off as soon as it is stopped. You may have to wait for up to a year before you notice any improvement. Ask your pharmacist for advice.

Using minoxidil
Apply the lotion to areas of hair loss using an applicator and spread it with your fingertips.

Disfigured or brittle nails

The most common cause of disfigured nails is a fungal infection. This usually affects toenails, particularly if your feet sweat a lot or you do not dry them properly after washing, although fingernails can also be infected if moisture gets trapped under artificial nails. The nail becomes thickened, crumbly, and white or yellow, and may grow misshapen or separate from the nail bed. Other nail problems include dry, hard, and brittle nails that are prone to splitting; white patches on the nails due to minor injuries; and fine vertical ridges on the nails, which are common in older people. In a few cases, nail changes indicate an underlying illness.

 See also Ringworm, p.48; Ingrown toenail, p.55.

 ## See your doctor first

Make an appointment to see your doctor if:

- You have a fungal infection of the nails
- You develop abnormalities such as curved or clubbed nails or pits on the nail surfaces

What you can do yourself

Use the following tips for fragile, brittle nails and to treat a fungal infection, alongside treatment prescribed by your doctor.

- Wash your hands after touching an infected nail. If your toenails are affected, don't walk barefoot around swimming pools, showers, and locker rooms; you may pass the infection on to others.

- Wear cotton socks rather than those made of synthetic fibers and change socks, pantyhose, or tights daily. Wear properly fitting shoes, made from natural materials that do not trap moisture. If your feet sweat, take your shoes off during the day, if possible, or wear open-toed sandals.

 - Practice good nail care to improve dry, brittle fingernails (*see* PRACTICAL TECHNIQUE, right).

- Wear cotton-lined rubber gloves to protect your hands when doing chores such as washing dishes or using household cleaning products.

- Try painting on a cosmetic nail hardener once a week. Don't wear artificial nails or nail polish.

- Very occasionally, buff vertical ridges on nails with a fine emery board to smooth them out. Be careful not to buff too much or you may thin the nail.

 ## PRACTICAL TECHNIQUE

Nail care This nail-care regimen will help keep your nails strong and healthy and reduce brittleness or splitting.

1 *Trim your nails regularly so that they are square at the sides and slightly rounded on the top. Trim hard or brittle nails after a bath or soak them in water first.*

2 *File your nails in one direction only, using gentle strokes from the side of the nail to its tip. Using a "sawing" motion with the file weakens the nail.*

3 *Don't have your cuticles removed during manicures; instead, soak your fingernails in warm water, then push the cuticles back gently with an orange stick.*

4 *At bedtime, rub a moisturizer into the cuticles and skin around the nails. Apply a moisturizer afterward whenever you wash your hands.*

 ## Seek further medical advice

See your doctor if your nail problems persist or if you develop any unexplained nail symptoms.

Nail biting

Many children and adolescents chew or bite on their fingernails, but most grow out of the habit eventually. Some people, however, continue to bite their nails in adult life, and the habit can be hard to break. You may find you bite your nails inadvertently when you are bored, or as a coping mechanism during times of stress or anxiety. In addition to being socially unappealing, nail biting transfers germs between your hands and your mouth and, if you chew the skin around your nails as well, it becomes susceptible to infections. You may also be ashamed of the appearance of your nails, particularly if biting makes them rough, torn, or split.

 ## See your doctor first

Make an appointment to see your doctor if:

- You or your child show other signs of anxiety such as hair pulling, or difficulty sleeping

What you can do yourself

Once you or your child have decided to stop nail biting, take these steps to help break the habit.

- Sit in front of a mirror and watch yourself biting your nails to see how unappealing it looks.

- Cut your nails short, and smooth them with a fine emery board so there are no ragged edges to chew. Put adhesive bandages around the tops of your fingers to keep from chewing loose bits of skin.

- Be aware of the times when you bite your nails and try to occupy your hands by fiddling with a pen, worry beads, or a piece of modeling clay.

- Chew sugar-free gum instead of your nails.

 - Paint an antinail-biting lotion on your nails (*see* DRUG REMEDIES, right).

- Reward yourself when your nails begin to look better. For example, have a professional manicure.

- Try having artificial nails fitted. They last for about 2 weeks, which may be long enough for you to break your nail-biting habit.

- Don't make your child feel guilty about nail biting. Try to find out if anything is causing anxiety and if there is something you can do to help.

- Use a star chart with your child. Reward each nail-biting-free day with a stick-on star and buy a small gift when the chart is complete.

 ### DRUG REMEDIES

Antinail-biting lotions (*see* p.179) have an extremely bitter taste that deters nibbling and acts as a reminder every time you start to bite. They can be used for children over 5, but work with your child, rather than forcing him or her to try one.

Using the lotion
Paint the lotion on like a nail polish once a day, paying particular attention to the top edge of the nails.

 ## Seek further medical advice

Arrange to see your doctor if:

- The skin around the nails becomes red and weepy or bleeds

Ingrown toenail

If your toe is painful, red, and swollen around the nail, the most likely cause is an ingrown nail. Big toes are most often affected. The nail begins to grow down into the skin on either side and the area becomes inflamed. Sometimes, the skin around the nail becomes infected, in which case there may be a discharge of pus. Cutting toenails incorrectly and wearing shoes that cramp the feet are the prime causes of this problem.

See your doctor first

Make an appointment to see your doctor if:

- Your toenail is inflamed and infected
- You have diabetes or poor circulation

What you can do yourself

In the early stages, when your toe is only slightly inflamed, you can treat it with the following measures. They may be enough to stop the problem from getting worse.

- Soak your foot twice a day for about 10 minutes in a bowl of warm water into which you have added 2–3 tablespoonfuls of salt. Put on a dry dressing to protect the toe. Wear open-toed sandals.

- Don't cut the nail until it has fully recovered.

- Don't use nail polish or nail-polish remover on the nail while it is inflamed.

PREVENTION

Preventing ingrown nails The simplest way to prevent ingrown toenails is to take good care of your feet.

- Wash your feet every day and dry them carefully.
- Don't wear shoes that squeeze or press on your toes. Avoid pointed styles and high heels.
- Change your socks, tights, or pantyhose daily and wear cotton socks rather than synthetics. Open-toed pantyhose and tights are available in some stores.
 - Make sure you cut your toenails correctly (*see* PRACTICAL TECHNIQUE, right).

PRACTICAL TECHNIQUE

How to cut toenails Adopt this nail-cutting routine to help prevent ingrown toenails. If you are elderly, or if you have diabetes or poor vision, seek specialist advice about nail care.

1 *Soften your toenails before you trim them by soaking them for 10 minutes in a bowl of warm water or in the bath. This will make them easier to cut, especially if they are tough or thick.*

2 *Use sharp nail scissors or clippers to cut your toenails straight across. Shape them so that they are rounded slightly at the tip, but don't cut into the corners since this encourages them to grow inward. Smooth the nail edges with a fine-textured file.*

3 *If a toenail is already growing into the skin, don't dig the scissors or clippers into the corner of the nail or try to push anything under the affected nail.*

Seek further medical advice

Arrange to see your doctor if:

- Your toe is getting worse or is not getting better after a few days of home treatment

EYE AND EAR PROBLEMS

Itchy eyes

Itchy eyes often look red, and there may also be irritation and a burning feeling. You may want to rub them continually. Anything that irritates the eyes, such as smoky atmospheres, dust, or infection, can produce itching, as can allergies such as hay fever or reactions to chlorinated swimming pools, cosmetics, or eyedrops. Sometimes, the edges of the eyelids can become infected. This condition, called blepharitis, results in sore, dry eyes with crusts on the eyelashes. Blepharitis is more common in people who have skin conditions such as dandruff. You may also develop itchy eyes occasionally if you wear contact lenses.

 See also **Dandruff**, p.49; **Dry eyes**, opposite page; **Conjunctivitis**, p.58; **Contact lens problems**, p.60.

 ## See your doctor first

Make an appointment to see your doctor to establish the cause of itchy eyes.

What you can do yourself

The following steps can help relieve the problem or be used with any treatment from your doctor.

● Avoid rubbing your eyes, since this can aggravate itching and can spread an infection.

● To help soothe allergic itching and irritation, use a cold compress. Soak a clean cloth (or cotton balls or pads) in cold water, wring it out, and lay it gently on your eyes for a few minutes. Repeat as needed, using a clean cloth or pads each time.

 ● Use artificial tears to help soothe itching due to allergies or to irritants such as dust and smoke (*see* DRUG REMEDIES, right).

● To find out if itching is caused by sensitivity to cosmetics, soap, or face or hair products, stop using them, then reintroduce items one by one to see if the problem returns. Throw away old eye makeup; don't keep mascara more than 6 months.

 ● If you have inflamed eyelids and crusty lashes, treat them with an eyelid-cleaning regimen (*see* PRACTICAL TECHNIQUE, right).

DRUG REMEDIES

Artificial tear drops and gels
containing hydroxypropyl methylcellulose keep the eyes moist and help relieve itching (*see* EYE LUBRICANTS, p.182). Don't wear contact lenses while using these.

PRACTICAL TECHNIQUE

Cleaning your eyelids Unless your doctor advises otherwise, try the following steps to help control blepharitis.

● Soak a clean washcloth in warm water, wring it out, then gently press it on your closed eyelid for about 5 minutes. This softens and loosens any crusts.
● Mix a little water with an equal amount of baby shampoo. Dip a cotton swab in the mixture, squeeze it out, and roll it along the edge of each eyelid to clean off debris and crusts. Rinse the eyelids with water, and dab them dry with a clean towel.
● Repeat, using a clean cloth, for the other eye.
● Clean your eyelids each morning and bedtime until they improve, then once daily to prevent a recurrence.

 ## Seek further medical advice

Arrange to see your doctor again if:

● Symptoms persist for more than 48 hours

Dry eyes

Dry eyes tend to develop when you are not producing enough tears or the tears are not lubricating the eye properly. Your eyes may feel irritated or gritty. People of any age can be affected, but older people, particularly women after menopause, are more susceptible. The problem is worsened by dry or windy weather, chlorinated swimming pools, and air conditioning or central heating. Diabetes, and certain medications such as antihistamines, can also cause dry eyes, as can inflammation of the eyelids (blepharitis).

 See also **Itchy eyes**, opposite page; **Conjunctivitis**, p.58; **Contact lens problems**, p.60.

 ## See your doctor first

Make an appointment to see your doctor to establish the cause of dry eyes.

What you can do yourself

Try the following measures to relieve the discomfort of dry eyes.

● Blink frequently, particularly when you are focusing on detailed work for long periods. Take frequent rests if you are working at a computer.

 ● For occasional dryness, use artificial tears to moisten your eyes (*see* DRUG REMEDIES, right).

 ● Try using a lubricating ointment to keep your eyes moist at night (*see* DRUG REMEDIES, right).

● In heated rooms, increase the humidity by using a humidifier, or place a bowl of water beside a radiator to keep the air moist.

● Drink 6–8 glasses of water a day. Cut down on coffee, tea, and cola, since these drinks contain caffeine, which can dehydrate you.

● Wear goggles when swimming.

● Avoid smoky or polluted environments, which could further irritate your eyes.

● Attach side shields to your glasses, especially in windy or dry conditions.

DRUG REMEDIES

Artificial tear drops and gels containing hydroxypropyl methylcellulose keep the eyes moist and can help relieve irritation (*see* EYE LUBRICANTS, p.182). Don't wear contact lenses while using these products.

Lubricating eye ointment (*see* EYE LUBRICANTS, p.182) is applied at bedtime to lubricate the eyes through the night. Lubricants are not usually recommended for use during the day as they may blur your vision. Ask your pharmacist to recommend an appropriate product.

Applying eye treatments
When using any eye treatment, apply it just inside your lower eyelid. Hold the end of the nozzle or dropper away from your eye to keep it clean.

 ## Seek further medical advice

Arrange to see your doctor again if:

● You often have dry, uncomfortable eyes
● You develop any other symptoms

Conjunctivitis

Red, itchy, gritty, and watery eyes are often due to conjunctivitis, inflammation of the membrane that covers the eye. You may also have a discharge that sticks your eyelids together. Infectious conjunctivitis tends to start in one eye and spread to the other. Allergic conjunctivitis may be seasonal, as with hay fever, or may be due to triggers such as dust mites and pet hair. It can also occur as a reaction to eye makeup or chemicals in eyedrops.

WARNING

Seek immediate medical help if:
● A red eye is associated with pain, blurred or reduced vision, or sensitivity to light

 See also **Hay fever**, p.80; **Wheezing**, p.103.

 ## See your doctor first

Arrange to see your doctor if you think you have conjunctivitis to establish the cause.

What you can do yourself

Once you know the cause of your attack of conjunctivitis, use the appropriate measures below to support any treatment from your doctor.

● Avoid wearing contact lenses if you have any form of conjunctivitis until you have been free of symptoms for at least 2 days.

● To avoid spreading conjunctivitis due to an infection, don't share towels, and change your towel and pillowcase every day. Try not to rub your eyes; if you do, wash your hands. Throw away eye makeup that you have been using recently.

 ● If your eyes are sticky or crusty each morning, clean them gently (*see* PRACTICAL TECHNIQUE, right).

● During the day, bathe your eyes with cool water to soothe them. This will also help to flush out pollen if you have allergic conjunctivitis. Tilt your head back and pour water into the corner of the eye, allowing it to wash over the eye.

● If conjunctivitis is due to allergy, use a cold compress to soothe irritation. Soak a clean cloth or cotton pad in cold water, wring it out, and place it over your eyes for a few minutes. Repeat as necessary, using a clean pad each time.

 ● For allergic conjunctivitis try antihistamine/ decongestant eyedrops (*see* DRUG REMEDIES, right).

 ### PRACTICAL TECHNIQUE

Cleaning sticky eyes Follow these steps to clean your eyes if they become sticky and crusted. (This usually happens overnight.) Treat one eye at a time to avoid spreading the infection from one eye to the other.

● Use a clean cotton ball dipped in warm water and, with the eye closed, gently wipe along your eyelids to remove any crusts.
● Wipe from the nose outward or the other way around, but keep wiping in the same direction.
● Repeat using a fresh cotton ball for the other eye.

 ### DRUG REMEDIES

Antihistamine/decongestant eyedrops (*see* p.178) contain the antihistamine pheniramine and the decongestant naphazalone. They act quickly to provide temporary relief of itchy, red, and watery eyes caused by allergic conjunctivitis.

 ## Seek further medical advice

Arrange to see your doctor again if:

● Conjunctivitis is not responding to treatment after a day or two
● You are using eyedrops but your symptoms are getting worse

Stye

A stye is a red bump on or inside the edge of your eyelid that swells up over a few days and becomes painful. The cause is an infection at the base of an eyelash. You may find it difficult to open your eye or feel as if you have something in your eye, especially when you blink. Your eye may also be watery and sensitive to light. The stye usually comes to a head and bursts, at which point the pain subsides, although some styes disappear without coming to a head.

Stye on the upper eyelid

 See also **Itchy eyes**, p.56; **Conjunctivitis**, opposite page.

What you can do yourself

A stye usually clears up by itself within a few days, but the following steps will help to minimize the pain and reduce the risk of spreading the infection.

- Don't rub your eye or squeeze the stye to release pus. Put a warm compress on it to bring it to a head (*see* PRACTICAL TECHNIQUE, right).

- Once the stye has burst, bathe your eyelid with warm water, then keep your eye clean and dry.

- Wash your hands regularly and avoid rubbing or touching the affected eye.

- Don't use eye makeup on the affected eye.

- Don't wear contact lenses while you have a stye.

 ## Seek medical advice

Arrange to see your doctor if:

- The stye hasn't healed, either on its own or with treatment, within a week
- The stye begins to spread to the skin on the surrounding eyelid
- You are getting recurrent styes

 ### PRACTICAL TECHNIQUE

Using a warm compress Soak a cotton pad or clean cloth in warm to hand-hot water, then squeeze it out and place it on your eyelid. Keep reapplying it for 10–15 minutes, rewarming the pad when it cools down. Repeat several times a day until the stye bursts.

Applying a compress
Use a clean pad for each session and keep rewarming it before holding it gently against your eyelid.

 ### PREVENTION

Preventing styes If you are prone to styes, use these hygiene measures to help prevent them.

- Wash your hands regularly and avoid touching your eyes. Always use your own washcloth and towel.
- Throw away old eye makeup, particularly liquids such as mascaras. Don't share makeup with other people. Remove makeup before you go to bed.
- If you use nondisposable contact lenses, be particularly careful about cleaning and storing them.

Contact lens problems

The most common causes of contact lens problems are lenses that fit badly, poor lens hygiene, sensitivity to cleaning solutions, and dusty, windy environments. If you wear lenses for too long, or get a piece of grit or dirt trapped under the lens, your eyes may become irritated, red, and watery. Sometimes a lens slips under the eyelid and needs to be retrieved and repositioned.

WARNING

Seek immediate medical help if:
- You have pain, blurred or reduced vision, or extreme sensitivity to light
- Your eye is very red

➤ *See also* **Dry eyes**, p.57.

What you can do yourself

The following steps will help reduce the risk of eye problems when you use contact lenses.

- If your eyes are irritated, take your contact lenses out for an hour or two to see if the symptoms ease. If they recur when you put the lenses back in, consult your optometrist or doctor.

- Try using lubricating eyedrops formulated for contact lens wearers (*see* DRUG REMEDIES, right).

- Unless you use continuous-wear lenses, don't wear your lenses longer than the period of time advised by your optometrist. If this is unavoidable, take them out from time to time to give your eyes a rest. Always remove lenses before going to bed, taking a nap, or swimming, bathing, or showering.

- Before handling lenses, wash your hands using an antibacterial or unperfumed soap and rinse them thoroughly. Clean and rinse reusable lenses every time you remove them using approved cleaners and storage solutions. Clean the lens case and air dry it. Never lick your lenses or use water to wet them.

- Ask your optometrist about using disposable contact lenses, which are worn for just one day and discarded. They don't need to be cleaned and sterilized and may be less likely to irritate your eyes.

- Be careful with makeup. Apply it after you put your lenses in, and don't use powder eye shadow or loose powder. Keep hairspray away from your eyes.

- Contact lenses can't really get "lost" in the eye, but sometimes a lens slips under the eyelid. Try this technique to get the lens back into position (*see* PRACTICAL TECHNIQUE, right).

DRUG REMEDIES

Lubricating and rewetting eyedrops containing sodium chloride (*see* EYE LUBRICANTS, p.182) make it easier to insert and remove lenses. Don't use other types of eyedrops without advice because some may damage your lenses.

PRACTICAL TECHNIQUE

If a lens has slipped under your eyelid, the following steps will help you retrieve it.

1 *First, squeeze 1–2 lubricating eyedrops into your eye. If your eye is dry, using drops may be enough to help the lens float back into its correct position.*

2 *If this doesn't work, close your eye, then guide the lens back into position by pressing lightly on your eyelid with one finger. This should encourage the lens to slide back down over the front of your eye.*

 Seek medical advice

See your doctor or optometrist promptly if:

- Eye irritation continues or there is a discharge
- You develop any new eye problems

Foreign object in the eye

If you get something in your eye, it can cause irritation, redness, watering, and blurred vision. In many instances, the foreign object is something tiny, such as an eyelash or a speck of dust or grit, and will wash out automatically as you blink and produce tears. If it remains floating on the white of your eye and you are sure there is no other injury, you can usually remove it yourself or get someone to remove it for you.

> ### WARNING
> Seek immediate medical attention if:
> ● An object sticks on or in the eye, or rests on the iris
> ● You think something entered your eye while you were using a power tool, or hammering or chiseling.

What you can do yourself

Take the following steps to remove a speck of dust or debris on the white of an eye.

● Don't rub the affected eye. Wash your hands thoroughly. If you are wearing contact lenses, remove them immediately.

● If you are treating someone else, sit the person in a well-lit place and check the eye for specks by gently pulling down the lower eyelid and asking him or her to look upward and then to the right and to the left. Repeat the procedure for the upper eyelid, pulling the eyelid up and asking the person to look down, right, and left. To check your own eye, sit in front of a mirror and pull your lower lid down and then the upper lid up.

● If you do find a speck of debris on the white of the eye, try flushing the eye with water (*see* PRACTICAL TECHNIQUE, right).

● If the speck has not been flushed out, try to lift it off the eye by lightly touching it with the edge of a clean, dampened handkerchief or tissue.

● If the speck is under the upper eyelid, grasp the upper lashes and pull the upper eyelid over the lower one to brush it out of the eye.

Seek medical advice

Arrange immediate medical help if:

● A foreign object cannot be removed easily
● You suffer pain, redness, extreme sensitivity to light, or blurred vision after you have removed a particle from your eye

PRACTICAL TECHNIQUE

Flushing out a foreign object
Use this procedure to flush a speck of debris out of your own or another person's eye.

● Treat another person's eye by putting a towel around his or her shoulders to catch runoff. Tilt the head to one side so that the affected eye is lower. Pour the water into the uppermost corner of the eye and let it drain out of the other side.
● Treat your own eye by filling a small glass, or eyebath if you have one, with water. Put a towel around your shoulders to catch runoff. Rest the rim of the glass or eye bath on the bone of the lower part of your eye socket. Keeping your eye open, tip your head back and pour in water to wash out the speck.

Flushing your eye
Pour the water directly into your eye, letting it drain freely onto the towel.

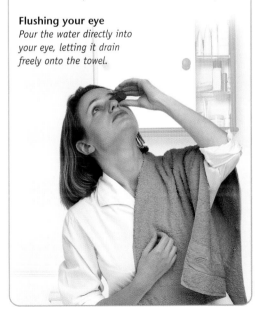

Black eye

A black eye is a bruise that develops around the eye, usually as a result of a direct blow to the eye. You may also get a black eye with other facial injuries because the skin around the eyes is delicate and easily bruised. Swelling, tenderness, and bleeding under the skin usually develop shortly after the injury. Later, the eyelids and surrounding area turn bluish black, and gradually fade to purple and then yellow as the bruise heals. Most black eyes disappear within 10–14 days.

WARNING

Seek medical help immediately if:
- You cannot see clearly and/or have blurred or double vision
- Your eye or eyelid is injured
- You lost consciousness, even for a short time

See your doctor first

Arrange to see your doctor urgently if:

- You are not certain how the black eye was caused or are concerned in any way about the condition of your eye

What you can do yourself

For a black eye caused by a minor injury, start using these home treatments as soon as possible to minimize bruising and discomfort.

- Apply an ice pack to the eye to reduce swelling and bleeding (*see* PRACTICAL TECHNIQUE, right).

- Keep your head raised on pillows at night to reduce the swelling.

- If necessary, take an analgesic (*see* DRUG REMEDIES, right) to relieve discomfort.

- Avoid contact sports until your eye has healed.

- Try not to blow your nose hard because it increases blood flow to the face and makes swelling around the eye worse.

Seek further medical advice

Arrange to see your doctor if:

- The black eye is not healing after a few days, becomes hot and swollen, or leaks pus
- There is any alteration in your vision
- You have persistent pain or headaches

PRACTICAL TECHNIQUE

Applying an ice pack Put something cold on a black eye as soon as possible to reduce swelling and bleeding under the skin.

- Use a bag of frozen peas or crushed ice wrapped in a wet towel, or a cloth soaked in cold water and wrung out. (If none are available, use a cold canned drink held lightly to the edge of the bruised area.)
- Hold the ice pack or cloth for 10–15 minutes without applying direct pressure to the eye.
- Reapply up to 8 times a day for the first 24–48 hours after the injury.

Treating your eye
Hold an ice pack or cold cloth gently on your eye, but don't press it hard against the skin.

DRUG REMEDIES

Analgesics Acetaminophen (*see* p.177) or ibuprofen (*see* p.185) will reduce the discomfort of a black eye. Avoid aspirin because it may prolong the bleeding that causes a black eye.

Earwax

Normally, earwax is produced in small amounts that protect the ear canal and disperse naturally. But if too much wax is produced, it can build up, become hard and dry, and block your ear canal. Using a cotton swab to clean the ears can cause wax to become impacted and contribute to blockages. A buildup of wax can cause hearing loss, discomfort, and a feeling of fullness in the ear. You may also notice itching, ringing (tinnitus), or dizziness. Wax buildup is more common in elderly people and in people who wear hearing aids.

 See also **Earache**, p.64; **Tinnitus**, p.67.

 ## See your doctor first

Arrange to see your doctor to confirm that there is a buildup of earwax, especially if you have had previous ear problems.

What you can do yourself

You only need to treat earwax if it is causing problems. You may be able to clear a buildup completely with the following measures. If you need to have your ears syringed by a doctor, these steps will also help to soften wax beforehand.

- Never use cotton swabs or push anything into your ear to clear wax. Aside from pushing wax farther into the ear canal, you may damage the ear canal lining, causing irritation and infection, or even damage the eardrum itself.

 - Treat your ears with something that will soften the wax. Try using olive oil or almond oil (*see* PRACTICAL TECHNIQUE, right).

 - Alternatively, try eardrops containing a wax solvent (*see* DRUG REMEDIES, right).

 ## Seek further medical advice

Arrange to see your doctor if:

- Your ear still feels as if it is blocked after you have tried self-help measures
- You develop an earache or a discharge of pus from the ear

 ### PRACTICAL TECHNIQUE

Softening wax in your ear Use a dropper bottle (ask your pharmacist) to apply olive oil or almond oil to the affected ear. If both ears are blocked, wait until one ear has cleared before treating the other, because the blockage may worsen temporarily as the wax softens.

- Allow half an hour for the olive or almond oil to warm to room temperature, or speed up the process by standing the bottle in warm water.
- Lying with the blocked ear upward, use the dropper to put 3–4 drops of warmed oil into the ear canal. Wait 10 minutes for them to be absorbed, then wipe off any excess oil.
- Repeat the process 3 times a day for 5 days.

Warming oils
Warm the olive or almond oil slightly by standing it in a bowl of hand-hot water for 10 minutes.

 ### DRUG REMEDIES

Earwax drops (*see* p.182) can be used to loosen and remove wax. They contain carbamide peroxide, which can sometimes irritate the ear canal. Ask your pharmacist for advice.

Earache

Pain in one or both ears and temporary hearing loss are often caused by a middle-ear infection, in which case you may also have a fever and feel generally ill. Sometimes, the eardrum bursts as a result of increased pressure and there is a discharge from the ear. An earache can also be caused by infection in the outer ear (swimmer's ear) or be associated with a throat or sinus infection or a tooth problem. You may also get a mild earache because of a buildup of mucus in your ear after a cold; during an attack of hay fever; or from pressure changes in the ear if you travel by plane or go diving.

 See also **Swimmer's ear**, opposite page; **Popping ears**, p.66; **Sinusitis**, p.79; **Earache (children)**, p.140.

 ## See your doctor first

Make an appointment to see your doctor if:

● You have a severe earache, develop a fever, or have a discharge from your ear

What you can do yourself

While following your doctor's advice, there are several measures you can take to relieve an earache or to treat a mild earache yourself.

 ● Take analgesics to reduce the discomfort (*see* DRUG REMEDIES, right).

● Sleep with your head raised on several pillows to reduce pressure in the middle ear.

 ● If your earache is due to a cold, try using decongestant nasal sprays or drops to help clear your nasal passages (*see* DRUG REMEDIES, right).

 ● Apply warmth to your ear to help relieve your earache (*see* PRACTICAL TECHNIQUE, right).

● Steam inhalation (*see* PRACTICAL TECHNIQUE, p.79) can help relieve congestion in the ear, nose, and sinuses. Putting a humidifier in the room may help.

● If your eardrum bursts, there may be a discharge. Keep your ear dry and arrange to see your doctor.

 ## Seek further medical advice

Arrange to see your doctor if:

● Your symptoms become more severe or do not subside within 24 hours of treatment

 ### DRUG REMEDIES

Analgesics Acetaminophen (*see* p.177) and ibuprofen (*see* p.185) will reduce discomfort, and will also reduce fever if you have an ear infection.

Decongestants (*see* p.181) in the form of nasal sprays or drops can help clear congestion in the nose, sinuses, and middle ear when you have a cold or allergy. Don't use a decongestant for more than 7 days continuously. If you use one for longer you may have a "rebound effect," with symptoms returning when you stop taking the drug.

 ### PRACTICAL TECHNIQUE

Using compresses You can make a warm compress by soaking a washcloth in warm water and squeezing it out. Hold the compress over the affected ear until the cloth cools down; then rewarm it. Alternatively, rest your ear on a heated pad or a covered hot-water bottle.

Applying warmth *Hold a warm, soft object (such as a warm compress) against your ear for about 20 minutes.*

Swimmer's ear

It's not only swimmers who get swimmer's ear (otitis externa). When you shower or wash your hair, trapped moisture can carry germs into the ear canal and cause an infection; the problem can also develop after ear syringing or if you work in warm and humid environments. Your ear may feel itchy and painful (particularly when you touch or pull your earlobe) and may feel blocked. There may also be a discharge of fluid from the ear. A scratch to the delicate lining of the ear canal, or a reaction to chemicals in eardrops or hair dyes, can also cause irritation and/or infection of the ear canal.

 See also Earwax, p.63.

 ## See your doctor first

Make an appointment to see your doctor if you think you might have swimmer's ear, to confirm the diagnosis.

What you can do yourself

Dealt with promptly, swimmer's ear normally clears up within a week or two. There are several things you can do to support treatment from your doctor.

- Your ear will be itchy, but don't scratch it.

- Don't use eardrops or treatments that have not been prescribed by your doctor.

- Keep your ear as dry as possible during treatment and for several days afterward. Take baths rather than showers. When you wash your hair, keep water out of your ears by placing cotton balls coated with petroleum jelly inside the entrance to each ear canal. Remove the pads afterward. Don't swim until the infection has cleared up.

- Hold a warm, dry washcloth or a covered hot-water bottle against your ear to help relieve the pain. Taking analgesics may also help (*see* DRUG REMEDIES, right).

- If you have a discharge, place a cotton ball over the outer part of your ear to absorb it. Make sure you change the cotton ball regularly. Don't try to clean your ear canal with cotton swabs, while you have an ear infection or at other times. They can damage your ear.

DRUG REMEDIES

Analgesics Take acetaminophen (*see* p.177) or ibuprofen (*see* p.185) to relieve any pain.

PREVENTION

Protecting your ears If you are prone to swimmer's ear, try these steps to help prevent it.

- Wear earplugs when you swim, and don't swim in polluted or dirty water.
- Always dry your ears carefully after washing your hair or showering. Tilt your head to one side and pull gently on each earlobe to help the water run out. Then use a hair dryer.
- Use unperfumed shampoos, and avoid hair dyes and styling products.

Drying safely
Use a hair dryer on a low heat and speed setting. Hold it 12 in (30 cm) from each ear.

 ## Seek further medical advice

Arrange to see your doctor again if:

- Your symptoms get worse or have not begun to respond to treatment after 2 days

Popping ears

The feeling of "popping ears" is common during air travel, scuba diving, or even when you travel up or down steep hills in a car. It is due to a difference in pressure between the outside environment and your middle ear, which makes your eardrum bulge and may cause pain, a muffled feeling, ringing in your ears, and temporary hearing loss. Normally, pressures are kept equal by air flowing in and out of the middle ear via the eustachian tubes, which link the middle ear to the nose and throat, but during rapid ascent or descent the tubes are too narrow to manage. Babies and young children have short, narrow tubes and are particularly prone to popping ears. Your ears are also more likely to pop if you have a blocked nose.

What you can do yourself

There are several steps that you can take to help equalize the pressure in your ears. The discomfort of popping ears usually disappears 3–5 hours after air pressure has stabilized.

- On a plane, chew gum or suck on a hard candy when you are ascending or descending rapidly.

- Swallowing frequently with your mouth open or yawning helps equalize the pressure.

- You can use a simple technique to unblock your ears (*see* PRACTICAL TECHNIQUE, right).

- If you are traveling with a baby, try breast-feeding or bottle-feeding while the plane is ascending or descending, or let your baby suck a pacifier. Give your baby plenty of fluids to drink during travel.

- If you are particularly susceptible to popping ears, take a decongestant before you travel (*see* DRUG REMEDIES, right).

- If you have a cold, an ear infection, or sinusitis, try to avoid air travel. If you must fly, use a decongestant. If you have hay fever when you fly, take an antihistamine (*see* DRUG REMEDIES, right). Don't scuba dive if you have any of these conditions.

 ## Seek medical advice

Arrange to see your doctor if:

- Your ears are very painful.
- Symptoms don't subside within 3–5 hours of returning to normal air pressure
- You have a discharge from your ear
- You have persistent hearing loss

PRACTICAL TECHNIQUE

Unblocking your ears Try the following action to relieve discomfort and unblock your ears. You may need to do this several times during ascent or descent.

- Begin by firmly pinching both of your nostrils closed with your index finger and thumb.
- Breathe in through your mouth. Then close your mouth, hold your nose tightly, and gently blow into your nostrils until your ears pop.

Blowing into your nostrils
Do not blow too hard, since you could damage your eardrums.

DRUG REMEDIES

Decongestants (*see* p.181), available as sprays and pills, shrink the membranes lining the nasal passages. When you fly, use a decongestant an hour before you take off, and repeat as necessary, following the instructions supplied with the product.

Antihistamines (*see* p.178) will relieve a blocked or runny nose caused by hay fever for the duration of your flight. Take a nonsedative antihistamine before traveling. Repeat as necessary, according to the instructions on the package label.

Tinnitus

If you suffer from tinnitus, you experience ringing, buzzing, or hissing noises that seem to be generated inside your ears or head with no external source for the sound. The noises, which may be continuous or may come and go, can affect sleep and concentration, and may make you depressed and anxious over time. Tinnitus is often linked to hearing loss, particularly in later life, or to repeated exposure to loud noise. Stress may make the problem worse. Air travel, high blood pressure, earwax buildup, certain inner ear problems, and some medications can all contribute to tinnitus. Sometimes, however, there is no apparent cause.

 See also Earwax, p.63; **Popping ears**, opposite page.

 ## See your doctor first

Make an appointment to see your doctor to confirm tinnitus and to find out whether a medicine you are taking, such as aspirin, is causing the problem or making it worse.

What you can do yourself

There isn't always a cure for tinnitus, but there are various things you can do that minimize its effects and make it easier to live with.

● Try using other sounds to distract you and mask the tinnitus. When you are trying to sleep, put on a fan, play soft music, listen to a ticking clock, or tune a radio so you can hear the interference hiss.

● Protect your ears with earplugs or earmuffs in noisy places or when you are using power tools such as a drill, since loud noise may make tinnitus worse.

● Cut down on caffeinated drinks such as coffee and cola. You should also avoid tonic water (which contains quinine), alcohol, and tobacco smoke. All of these substances make tinnitus worse.

● A low-salt diet may be helpful. Add less salt when cooking and use herbs and spices instead.

 ● Using ginkgo may help reduce tinnitus (*see* NATURAL REMEDIES, right).

● If stress makes your tinnitus worse, get regular exercise and try using measures to reduce stress in your life (*see* STRESS, pp.20–21).

● If you have persistent tinnitus, joining a support group for sufferers can be a good way to share problems and discuss solutions.

 ### NATURAL REMEDIES

Ginkgo preparations (see p.183) are made from the leaves of the maidenhair tree and have been shown to help some people with tinnitus. They are available in pharmacies and health stores, but you need to consult your doctor before using them. Follow the dosage instructions carefully.

Taking ginkgo
You will probably have to take a ginkgo supplement for 4–6 weeks to find out if it is going to be helpful.

 ## Seek further medical advice

Arrange to see your doctor again if:

● Your tinnitus gets worse, or does not respond to the treatment advised by your doctor or to the self-help measures described above
● You also feel dizzy or sick
● You develop hearing loss

Foreign object in the ear

If something becomes lodged in your ear it can cause irritation, and can result in temporary hearing loss if it blocks your ear canal. A sharp object can damage your eardrum. Young children sometimes push small items such as beads or bits of paper into their ears. Unless you see them doing it, you may not be aware of a problem until they complain of pain in the ear, have a discharge from it, or are unable to hear properly. Adults sometimes get cotton stuck inside the ear canal while cleaning their ears (a practice that is not recommended). Occasionally, insects get lodged in the ears; this can be alarming, especially for a child.

 See also Earwax, p.63.

 ## See your doctor

Make an urgent appointment to see your doctor if an object does not fall out of the ear by itself or if you cannot remove an insect using the measures below.

What you can do yourself

There are limited steps that you can take to deal with an object or insect in the ear; if they don't work, see your doctor.

- Try tilting the ear downward and shaking it gently to see if the object or insect falls out.

- If there is an insect in the ear, try to stay calm. Tilt the affected ear upward and wait to see if the insect crawls out by itself. If it doesn't, try floating it out with water (*see* PRACTICAL TECHNIQUE, right).

- Never try to remove something from the ear by probing with fingers, tweezers, or a cotton swab, even if you can see it. You are likely to push the object further into the ear, and may damage the lining of the ear and/or the eardrum.

 ## Seek further medical advice

Arrange to see your doctor urgently if, after removing an object:

- There is still a feeling of something in the ear
- Your hearing is impaired
- Your ear is painful or there is a discharge

PRACTICAL TECHNIQUE

Removing an insect from the ear You may be able to remove an insect from the ear by floating it out. If the insect is in your own ear, get someone to help you. (Don't use water to remove anything other than an insect, because some objects may swell up and become more difficult to remove.)

- Have some lukewarm water ready and a dropper.
- Ask the person to lie down with the affected ear upward and to keep very still.
- Trickle water into the ear using the dropper. This should cause the insect to float out of the ear.
- Tilt the head downward to let any remaining water drain away.
- If the insect does not float out, don't make further attempts to remove it. Seek medical help.

Floating out an insect
A child may be frightened at the thought of having an insect in the ear, so calm him or her down first. Ask the child to lie very still while you drop water into the ear.

MOUTH, NOSE, AND THROAT PROBLEMS

Chapped or cracked lips

Almost everyone gets dry, chapped lips occasionally. Lips are sensitive to sunlight, and dry out easily in cold, windy weather and in heated rooms. The problem is worsened if you lick your lips habitually. These same conditions can cause cracks in the skin folds at the corners of the mouth where moisture gathers. The skin may be sore, and you may have a burning sensation when you open your mouth. The area may become weepy, and a yeast infection may develop. Elderly people, particularly those who have worn dentures or teeth missing, are prone to the problem, as are babies who drool or overuse a pacifier. Underlying illnesses such as anemia can contribute. An allergic reaction, for example to cosmetics, may also cause sore lips.

What you can do yourself

Just a few days of care and attention will help improve the condition of dry, sore lips and related problems. Combine the treatment with preventive measures to protect your lips.

- If you have cracked or sore lips, put some petroleum jelly on them or try a cream or balm from your pharmacist. Before you go out in cold, dry weather, apply a moisturizing lip salve on and around your lips (*see* DRUG REMEDIES, right).

- If you suspect that your lip symptoms are an allergic reaction, throw away any toothpastes, cosmetics, and lip products that you have been using. Introduce a new toothpaste and new lip products one by one and watch for reactions.

- Avoid acidic or spicy foods or drinks that may "burn" sore skin.

- Drink plenty of water (at least 6–8 glasses a day), particularly when the heat is on.

- Try to stop licking your lips.

- See your dentist if you have teeth problems: for example, if your dentures do not fit well.

DRUG REMEDIES

Lip creams, balms, and salves

(*see* p.186) moisturize and soothe sore, chapped lips and cracked corners of the mouth. Use a lip salve with a minimum sun protection factor (SPF) of 15 in sunshine and one with an SPF of 25 or higher at high altitudes. Most contain moisturizers and are water resistant. Ask your pharmacist for advice.

Protecting your lips
Reapply lip balm or salve frequently, especially in cold, windy weather and at high altitudes.

Seek medical advice

Arrange to see your doctor if:

- The area of skin becomes red and weepy and there is a discharge
- The cracked skin is getting worse or is not getting better after about 10 days
- You regularly get cracked mouth corners

Cold sore

Cold sores begin with tingling near the mouth, followed by a cluster of small, painful blisters. These sores burst and crust over, but normally heal within about 10 days. They are caused by the herpes simplex virus, which lies dormant in the body after a first infection. Triggers such as colds and the flu, fatigue, stress, menstruation, cold, wind, or strong sunshine can reactivate the virus, causing another cold sore.

Cold sore on lip

 ## See your doctor first

Make an appointment to see your doctor promptly if you are developing a cold sore in or near your eye.

What you can do yourself

You can't get rid of the cold sore virus, but the following measures will reduce the time a cold sore lasts and help prevent flare-ups.

- As soon as you notice tingling, apply a small ice pack (a packet of frozen peas or crushed ice in a plastic bag, wrapped in a washcloth) to the area, for about 5–10 minutes every half hour.

- Take an analgesic if your cold sore is very uncomfortable (*see* DRUG REMEDIES, right).

- Apply petroleum jelly to the affected area to help prevent cracking or bleeding.

- Try using tea tree oil (*see* NATURAL REMEDIES, right) to soothe the pain and help your sore heal.

- Cold sores are contagious. While you have symptoms, avoid close contact such as kissing and don't share towels, cups and glasses, or razors.

- After touching a sore, wash your hands to avoid spreading the virus. Don't pick or squeeze sores.

- If sunlight triggers cold sores, use sunscreen or a lip balm with sunscreen when you spend time in the sun (*see* DRUG REMEDIES, p.69).

- If stress or fatigue are triggers, get plenty of sleep, and try deep breathing and muscle relaxation exercises (*see* PRACTICAL TECHNIQUES, pp.20–21).

- If you have recurrent cold sores, your doctor may prescribe acyclovir cream (*see* DRUG REMEDIES, right).

DRUG REMEDIES

Analgesics such as acetaminophen (*see* p.177) or ibuprofen (*see* p.185) can help to ease the discomfort of a cold sore.

Acyclovir cream, which is available by prescription, acts against the herpes virus and can reduce the duration and severity of a cold sore. Apply as directed by your doctor at the first sign of tingling or burning.

Using acyclovir
Apply acyclovir cream thinly to the area as soon as you notice the signs that a cold sore is developing.

NATURAL REMEDIES

Tea tree oil (*see* p.189), which can be applied as a roll-on or dabbed directly onto a cold sore, may help the blisters dry out and heal more quickly.

 ## Seek further medical advice

Arrange to see your doctor if:

- **The sore is getting worse, or is not getting better after about 10 days despite treatment**
- **You have frequent cold sores**

Mouth ulcer

Common mouth ulcers start with burning pain or soreness, then a shallow, grayish white pit with a red border develops. The ulcers tend to recur, but are not contagious. They are more likely to develop if you are run down or stressed. Some women get them before a menstrual period. Badly fitting dentures or careless toothbrushing can also cause them. Rarely, an ulcer in the mouth may be due to cancer.

Common mouth ulcer on gum

 ## See your doctor first

Make an appointment to see your doctor if:

- You also feel sick and/or have a fever
- Many ulcers develop at the same time
- You have had a mouth ulcer for longer than 2 weeks and/or it is getting bigger

What you can do yourself

A common mouth ulcer normally disappears within a week or two without treatment, but it can be very uncomfortable. Try the following measures to reduce pain and help the ulcer heal more quickly.

- Eat soft, soothing foods, such as yogurt, ice cream, and custard. Sip cool water or other cooling drinks through a straw.

- Avoid any food or drink that will irritate your mouth and aggravate your ulcer, such as citrus fruits and drinks; coffee; salty or spicy foods; hard foods such as nuts, potato chips, and toast; and very hot foods or drinks.

- Clean your teeth using a soft toothbrush.

 - Use an antiseptic mouthwash (*see* DRUG REMEDIES, right). Alternatively, make a salt-water mouthwash by dissolving half a teaspoon of salt in 1 cup (250 ml) of warm water and use it several times a day. Swish the mouthwash around your mouth for about 30 seconds, then spit it out.

 - Ease pain by applying preparations that contain a local anesthetic (*see* DRUG REMEDIES, right).

DRUG REMEDIES

Antiseptic mouthwashes Rinsing your mouth with an antiseptic mouthwash (*see* MOUTH AND THROAT TREATMENTS, p.187) reduces the risk of a secondary infection and will help your mouth ulcer heal.

Local anesthetics The local anesthetic benzocaine (*see* MOUTH AND THROAT TREATMENTS, p.187) helps to numb a mouth ulcer and provide temporary relief of pain. Local anesthetic preparations are available as liquids to dab on, gels, and lozenges. Using a local anesthetic regularly may increase irritation. Do not use for more than 7 days unless directed to by your doctor or dentist.

 ## Seek further medical advice

Arrange to see your doctor if:

- You have severe pain that is not controlled by the measures described above
- You have difficulty swallowing
- The ulcer has not healed within 2 weeks and/or it is getting bigger
- You have recurrent mouth ulcers

Bad breath

Unpleasant-smelling breath, known medically as halitosis, is usually due to poor mouth hygiene. Particles of food left in the mouth and between the teeth are broken down by bacteria and cause an offensive smell. Particular foods and drinks, such as garlic and beer, can make your breath smell. Bad breath also tends to occur when your mouth is dry, and is often a problem right after waking up. Other possible causes include a sinus or throat infection, diabetes, lung disease, or a weight-loss diet.

What you can do yourself

The following simple measures will help you tackle bad breath. Make them part of your daily routine.

- Brush your teeth before going to bed and when you get up. Brush your tongue as well. Use a soft-bristled brush and a fluoride toothpaste, and make sure you rinse thoroughly afterward.

- Floss your teeth once a day to remove plaque (*see* PRACTICAL TECHNIQUE: ORAL HYGIENE, p.74).

- If you wear dentures, take them out at night and clean them thoroughly, as recommended by your dentist. You should also clean removable braces and attached dental appliances as advised by your orthodontist.

- Make sure you eat breakfast because it stimulates saliva, which helps to wash away bacteria that may have built up overnight. Fruit and vegetables also stimulate saliva, so include plenty of them in your daily diet.

- Take a toothbrush to work or school so you can brush after meals. If you can't clean your teeth between meals, chew sugar-free gum, which encourages saliva flow.

- Mouthwashes and breath fresheners have only a temporary effect but can be a useful short-term measure (*see* DRUG REMEDIES, right).

- Avoid spicy or strong-smelling foods. When you can't avoid these foods, finish the meal with some fruit to freshen the mouth.

- Drink at least 6–8 glasses of water each day. Avoid alcohol, tea, and coffee; they have a dehydrating effect that can encourage bad breath.

- Don't smoke. Cigarettes are a major cause of bad breath.

DRUG REMEDIES

Mouthwashes (*see* MOUTH AND THROAT TREATMENTS, p.187) usually contain flavorings and extracts such as menthol to freshen the breath. They may also contain fluoride to protect against tooth decay and gum disease. Don't give mouthwashes to children because they could easily swallow them.

Breath fresheners (*see* MOUTH AND THROAT TREATMENTS, p.187), in the form of sprays and little strips that dissolve on the tongue, can be an effective short-term remedy for bad breath. They mask the breath with a pleasant (usually minty) smell; the effect usually lasts for about 20 minutes.

Breath freshening
Use a breath-freshener spray as a temporary measure to mask lingering smells after a spicy meal.

✚ Seek medical advice

Arrange to see your doctor if:

- You have tried the above measures for about a week and bad breath persists
- You also have a toothache, or inflamed or bleeding gums
- You feel generally unwell and think this may be contributing to bad breath

Sore mouth or tongue

There are several possible causes for a sore mouth or tongue. The lining of your mouth can become irritated and inflamed by hot, spicy foods or hot drinks, or because you overuse mouthwashes, drink heavily, or smoke. Your tongue may be tender and have a smooth, red appearance, and your sense of taste may be altered. You may also get a sore mouth if you bite your tongue or cheek accidentally, or if you have rough or broken teeth or badly fitting dentures. Other causes include common mouth ulcers, gum disorders, and mouth infections such as yeast. In rare cases, a sore mouth is caused by a more serious illness.

See also **Mouth ulcer**, p.71; **Bleeding gums**, p.74.

 ## See your doctor first

Make an appointment to see your doctor if:

- You have signs of an infection, such as white patches inside your mouth
- You feel lethargic, are not eating well, and/or are losing weight
- Your mouth and eyes are persistently dry

What you can do yourself

Use the following home treatments to soothe an irritated mouth and tongue:

- Drink 6–8 glasses of fluid a day. Cool drinks and popsicles are soothing. Don't drink alcohol or smoke – both can irritate your mouth.

- Try using a homemade mouthwash (*see* NATURAL REMEDIES, right). Avoid mouthwashes that contain alcohol because they may cause further irritation.

- Don't give up brushing your teeth, just do it gently using a very soft toothbrush.

- Eat small, frequent meals of soft foods, such as pudding, mashed potato and gravy, yogurt, and custard. Avoid salty, spicy foods, coarse foods such as toast, and acidic fruit juices.

- Try using a pain-relieving mouth treatment (*see* DRUG REMEDIES, right).

- If you have a dry mouth, use sugar-free chewing gum to stimulate saliva flow.

- See your dentist if you have rough or broken teeth, or if your dentures don't fit properly.

 ### NATURAL REMEDIES

Soothing mouthwash Dissolve half a teaspoon of baking soda (*see* p.179) or salt in 1 cup (250 ml) of warm water, and use this to rinse your mouth regularly during the day, especially after eating. Swish the mouthwash around your mouth for about 30 seconds before spitting it out.

 ### DRUG REMEDIES

Pain-relieving mouth treatments (*see* MOUTH AND THROAT TREATMENTS, p.187) can help to relieve soreness. Some rinses, lozenges, and sprays reduce pain and inflammation, while others contain a local anesthetic that numbs sore areas. However, using anesthetic preparations regularly may increase irritation. Ask your pharmacist for advice before giving mouth treatments to a child.

 ## Seek further medical advice

Arrange to see your doctor if:

- The soreness becomes worse, or does not subside after a few days of using the self-help measures described here

Bleeding gums

Bleeding from the gums is usually a sign of gum inflammation (gingivitis). Healthy gums are pale and firm, but diseased gums may become purplish red, swollen, and shiny, and bleed when you brush your teeth. Your breath may smell unpleasant. The cause is usually a buildup of plaque (a deposit formed from food particles, saliva, and bacteria) at the base of the teeth due to poor oral hygiene. Bleeding gums can also be due to vigorous brushing or poorly fitting dentures. You may be prone to them during pregnancy or if you take certain drugs.

 See also Bad breath, p.72.

See your dentist or doctor first

Arrange to see your dentist or doctor if:

- You have a toothache or loose teeth
- You bruise easily and feel tired and weak
- You are taking a prescribed medicine, such as an anticoagulant, that may cause bleeding gums. Don't stop taking prescribed medicine without consulting your doctor

What you can do yourself

Use these measures to help your gums heal and prevent more serious damage to gums and teeth.

- If bleeding is profuse, try pressing a piece of gauze or cotton ball soaked in ice-cold water on your gums for a few minutes.

 - Practice good oral hygiene (*see* PRACTICAL TECHNIQUE, right). Brush your teeth gently using a new, soft-bristled brush, making sure you don't scratch your gums. Use dental tape or floss, or a tapered interdental brush (which looks like a tiny bottlebrush), to clean between your teeth.

- Don't use toothpicks to clean between your teeth, because they can injure your gums.

- Stop smoking, because tobacco smoke aggravates bleeding gums.

Seek further medical advice

Arrange to see your dentist or doctor if:

- Your gums are still bleeding after you have tried the above measures for 7–10 days
- You have any other symptoms

PRACTICAL TECHNIQUE

Oral hygiene The following oral hygiene routine helps reduce the risk of gum disease and prevent tooth decay. Brush your teeth at least twice a day, and replace your toothbrush every 2–3 months. Clean between your teeth with dental floss or tape. There are many types available; tape may be more comfortable for your gums.

1 *Brush your teeth before going to bed and when you get up in the morning or after breakfast. Use fluoride toothpaste and a small, soft-bristled brush. Brush all the surfaces of your teeth, especially where they meet the gums, using short, vertical or circular strokes.*

2 *Use dental tape or floss once a day to get rid of plaque between your teeth and at the gum line. Wind a piece around one finger of each hand. Keeping it taut, move it up and down the side of a tooth, going slightly below the gum line. Repeat, using fresh pieces, for every tooth.*

Toothache and sensitive teeth

A toothache can range from a mild ache to a continuous throbbing pain. Tooth decay, usually due to poor dental hygiene, is the most common cause, but pain in the teeth can also be due to gum disease, a cracked tooth, or jaw problems. Teens and adults may have pain from wisdom teeth emerging. Your teeth may become sensitive to hot or cold or to brushing if the enamel that protects them becomes worn or cracked, or if your gums recede and expose the inner layers of the teeth.

WARNING

See your dentist immediately or go to an emergency room if you have severe, continuous pain when you bite; fever; foul-smelling breath; and/or a swollen face. You may have a tooth abscess.

 ## See your dentist first

Make an appointment to see your dentist if you are suffering from toothache.

What you can do yourself

Take the following steps to relieve a painful tooth while you are waiting for an appointment with your dentist, or to reduce general sensitivity in your teeth.

● Avoid eating or drinking anything very hot or very cold if this makes the pain worse. Some people, however, find that sucking on an ice cube in the area of the toothache brings relief. Stop if the tooth becomes more painful.

● Rinse your mouth thoroughly with a salt water mouthwash. To make it, mix a teaspoon of salt in a cup of warm water.

 ● Try applying oil of cloves to a painful tooth (*see* NATURAL REMEDIES, right).

 ● Take an analgesic such as acetaminophen or ibuprofen (*see* DRUG REMEDIES, right).

● Use dental floss or tape to remove any food debris trapped between your teeth. Gently clean either side of the painful tooth.

● If you have sensitive teeth, brush your teeth gently using toothpaste formulated for sensitive teeth. After brushing, massage a little toothpaste into your gums and leave it on overnight.

 ● Establish a good oral hygiene routine to prevent further tooth decay (*see* PRACTICAL TECHNIQUE, opposite page).

 ### NATURAL REMEDIES

Oil of cloves (*see* p.187) is a traditional remedy from your pharmacist that may help to soothe an aching tooth. Put a few drops of the oil on a cotton ball, place it on the painful tooth, and bite down gently. Be careful to keep the oil off your tongue because it may burn a little.

Clove oil
The oil is distilled from cloves and is antiseptic and anesthetic, which makes it useful for relieving a toothache.

 ### DRUG REMEDIES

Analgesics that can relieve the pain of a toothache include acetaminophen (*see* p.177) and ibuprofen (*see* p.185).

● For a child, give acetaminophen (*see* p.177) or ibuprofen (*see* p.185), both available as liquid medicine. Make sure you ask your pharmacist to recommend an appropriate product for your child.

Knocked-out tooth

Teeth are often knocked out during accidents, particularly during contact sports such as football. The front teeth are the most vulnerable. If you lose one of your permanent teeth, you may be able to save it by replacing it quickly and getting emergency help. If a tooth is replaced in the socket within about 30 minutes of being knocked out, there is a 90 percent chance it will be saved, and the chances are still good for up to 2 hours. A broken tooth, however, cannot be saved. Children sometimes lose baby teeth in a fall, but these will be replaced eventually by permanent teeth so there is no need to replace them.

 ## Seek immediate medical advice

If your tooth has been knocked out or loosened by an injury, see your dentist or go to an emergency room as soon as possible. If a child loses a baby tooth, it is important to see a dentist to check for possible damage to the mouth or gums.

What you can do yourself

Immediately after the accident, take the following steps to maximize the chances of saving your tooth. Replacing the tooth is the best option, but if you can't do this, you must make sure that the tooth does not dry out while you seek medical help.

- Find the missing tooth and pick it up by the top (the crown), not the root. Do not rub or scrape it to remove dirt or any tissue fragments attached to it. Rinse it gently in a glass of tap water, but don't hold it under running water.

- Put the tooth back in its socket (*see* PRACTICAL TECHNIQUE, right).

- If you can't replace a permanent tooth in its socket, tuck it under your tongue or inside your cheek. Alternatively, place the tooth in a glass of milk or some of your own saliva.

- If a child has lost a baby tooth and the socket is bleeding, rinse out his or her mouth with water and place a wad of tissue or gauze in the socket. Your child should bite down on it to stop the bleeding.

 ### PRACTICAL TECHNIQUE

Replacing a tooth Whenever possible, you should try to save a permanent tooth by replacing it quickly in the socket. Don't attempt to do this, however, if you are concerned that the victim may swallow or choke on the loose tooth.

1 *Wash your hands thoroughly or put on disposable gloves, if available. Pick up the tooth by the crown and hold it firmly. Check that it is the right way around before pushing it firmly into the socket. Do this even if the socket is bleeding.*

2 *Hold the tooth in place with your fingers, or put a piece of gauze on the tooth and bite down gently on it. Go to a hospital emergency room or to an emergency dentist for immediate treatment.*

Blocked or runny nose

If you have a runny or blocked nose, you feel stuffed up, may lose your sense of taste and smell, and may only be able to breathe through your mouth. You may cough at night because of mucus dripping down the back of your throat. If your blocked nose is due to a cold or sinus infection, you may also have a thick yellowish green discharge from your nose. A blocked or runny nose can also be caused by allergies to substances such as pollen, dust mites, pet dander (flakes of skin), and mold. Symptoms can occur at any time or be seasonal, as with hay fever.

 See also **Common cold**, p.78; **Sinusitis**, p.79; **Hay fever**, p.80; **Coughing**, p.102.

What you can do yourself

Try the following home treatments to help relieve your blocked or runny nose.

 ● Drink at least 8 glasses a day of clear fluids such as water, herbal tea, and clear soup. Hot drinks help loosen mucus if your nose is blocked, as will saline nose drops (*see* DRUG REMEDIES, right).

● Try a steam inhalation, or run hot water into the bath or shower and inhale the steam (*see* PRACTICAL TECHNIQUE: STEAM INHALATION, p.79).

 ● Remedies containing essential oils may help relieve a stuffy nose (*see* NATURAL REMEDIES, right).

 ● If you have a blocked nose due to a cold, try a decongestant nasal spray (*see* DRUG REMEDIES, right).

● If your nose is sore from blowing it, apply some petroleum jelly around your nostrils to protect them.

 ● To treat a blocked or runny nose caused by an allergy, use cromolyn sodium nasal spray and/or an oral antihistamine (*see* DRUG REMEDIES, right).

● Avoid smoke and dust; they can irritate the lining of your nose and worsen symptoms.

 ## Seek medical advice

Arrange to see your doctor if:

● Symptoms have not begun to clear up using the measures described here
● You develop new symptoms
● You are using medications continually to relieve your blocked or runny nose

NATURAL REMEDIES

Essential oils (*see* p.182) such as menthol, eucalyptus, or camphor, are traditional treatments for a blocked nose. Try sucking lozenges containing menthol, or putting a few drops of an essential oil on a tissue and inhaling it. Use a menthol chest rub at night if you are having difficulty sleeping.

DRUG REMEDIES

Saline nose drops (*see* p.188) can be bought from your pharmacist, or you can make your own by dissolving half a teaspoon of salt in 1 cup (250 ml) of lukewarm water. Apply them using a dropper, 2–4 times a day.

Decongestants (*see* p.181), available as nasal sprays or drops, quickly relieve a blocked nose by reducing swelling and congestion in the tissues lining the nose. They also lessen mucus production. They should not, however, be used for more than 7 days, otherwise they may make you feel more blocked when you stop using them.

Cromolyn sodium nasal spray (*see* p.181) helps to prevent or relieve a runny nose caused by allergies such as hay fever and dust mites. It must be used continuously

Antihistamines (*see* p.178), in the form of pills or liquids, usually work within 1 hour. You can use them to relieve a runny nose due to allergies, but they are not so effective for a blocked nose. They can be taken regularly or only as needed – for example, if you are visiting a house with pets.

Common cold

Colds are common infections of the nose and throat that can be caused by more than 200 different, highly contagious viruses. You are likely to pick up at least one or two colds a year, usually from the coughs and sneezes of infected people. Children are even more susceptible because they have not built up immunity to cold viruses. Typical symptoms are a blocked or runny nose, sneezing, reduced sense of taste and smell, a sore throat, a dry cough, headache, and mild fever. Colds can be more serious in babies and elderly people.

 See also **Blocked or runny nose**, p.77; **Sore throat**, p.81; **Headache**, p.85.

What you can do yourself

Most people recover from a cold within a week, but there are things you can do to make yourself feel better in the meantime.

- Drink at least 8 glasses of warm liquids a day such as herbal teas and clear soups. Avoid tea and coffee. To relieve a sore throat, make a warm honey and lemon drink (*see* NATURAL REMEDIES, p.30).

- Take an analgesic or a cold remedy to relieve discomfort (*see* DRUG REMEDIES, right).

- Try a steam inhalation to clear a stuffy nose (*see* PRACTICAL TECHNIQUE, opposite page). You can also use saline nose drops (*see* DRUG REMEDIES, opposite page) or a decongestant (*see* DRUG REMEDIES, right).

- Use paper tissues rather than handkerchiefs to blow your nose. If your nose is sore, try tissues with soothing ingredients such as aloe vera.

- Antihistamines may help to relieve a runny nose and reduce sneezing (*see* DRUG REMEDIES, right).

- You may be able to speed your recovery by taking zinc, and relieve the worst symptoms of a cold with echinacea (*see* NATURAL REMEDIES, right).

- Do not smoke, and avoid smoky environments.

Seek medical advice

Arrange to see your doctor if:

- Your cold persists for more than **10 days**
- You develop a severe sore throat or high fever, or cough up yellow or green mucus
- You have an earache or face pain and/or a greenish yellow nasal discharge

DRUG REMEDIES

Analgesics Acetaminophen (*see* p.177), aspirin (*see* p.179), or ibuprofen (see p.185) can help to relieve headache, fever, and a sore throat.

CAUTION: Children should not use aspirin before a doctor is consulted about Reye's syndrome (see p.179).

Cold and flu remedies (*see* p.180) contain analgesics, decongestants, and antihistamines to relieve a range of symptoms. Don't use them with other analgesics because of the risk of overdose.

Decongestants (*see* p.181) in the form of nasal sprays or drops containing phenylephrine or oxymetazoline can help clear a blocked nose.

Antihistamines (*see* p.178) can help clear up a runny nose and sneezing, although they tend to dry out the nasal passages.

NATURAL REMEDIES

Zinc lozenges (*see* p.189), taken early on in a cold, may help shorten the illness. Occasionally, they cause a bad taste in the mouth and mild nausea.

Echinacea (*see* p.182), taken as a tincture or capsules, can help reduce cold symptoms and speed recovery.

Using echinacea
The herb is most effective when taken at the start of a cold.

Sinusitis

Sinusitis is an inflammation of the membranes lining the sinuses, which are air-filled pockets located behind the nose, cheeks, and forehead. It causes pain and tenderness around the eyes and cheeks; a stuffy and/or runny nose; and, sometimes, aching in the upper teeth and jaw. You may also have a foul taste in your mouth and feel feverish. Sinusitis is usually a complication of an infection such as a cold or the flu. People who swim or dive regularly may be more susceptible than usual to the problem.

WARNING

Seek immediate medical help if you also develop severe headaches, vomiting, and fever.

See your doctor first

Make an appointment to see your doctor if you think you may have sinusitis, to confirm the diagnosis and get advice on treatment.

What you can do yourself

You can do several things to relieve the "heavy-headed" feeling of sinusitis and speed your recovery.

● Put a warm, moist washcloth over your nose to relieve pain, or use steam inhalation up to 3–4 times a day to reduce congestion (*see* PRACTICAL TECHNIQUE, right).

● If you are in pain or have a fever, take an analgesic (*see* DRUG REMEDIES, right).

● Drink at least 8 glasses of warm fluids a day.

● Decongestants may help clear your nose. Alternatively, try using saline nose drops to loosen mucus. (*See* DRUG REMEDIES, right.)

● Blow your nose gently.

● Get plenty of rest. Sleep with your head raised. Sleeping on your side may make breathing easier.

● Try to avoid spending time in cold, polluted, or smoky atmospheres.

Seek further medical advice

Arrange to see your doctor if your sinusitis has not begun to clear up after a few days.

PRACTICAL TECHNIQUE

Steam inhalation This helps loosen mucus in the nose, throat, and sinuses. Children should only use steam inhalations if supervised by an adult.

● Fill a bowl one-third full with hot, but not boiling, water. You can add eucalyptus oil, pine oil, or menthol (*see* ESSENTIAL OILS, p.182) to make it smell pleasant.

● Lean forward, cover your head and the bowl with a towel, and gently inhale the steam. If your nose is blocked, breathe through your mouth until your nose clears.

Inhaling steam
Breathe in and out through your nose for several minutes.

DRUG REMEDIES

Analgesics, such as acetaminophen (*see* p.177) and ibuprofen (*see* p.185), will help relieve pain around the eyes and the cheeks and will also reduce the fever that can accompany sinusitis.

Decongestants (*see* p.181) help reduce swelling inside the nose and sinuses.

Saline nose drops (*see* p.188) can be used up to 6 times a day to help loosen mucus in the nasal passages.

Hay fever

Hay fever is caused by an allergy to pollen or mold. When pollen grains or mold spores get into your eyes, nose, or airways, they cause symptoms such as sneezing; a runny or blocked nose; itching in your eyes, nose, and the roof of your mouth; watery, red eyes; and a cough. You may also develop wheezing. Symptoms can develop at any time from early spring to early fall, depending on which pollens or molds trigger the allergy. Hay fever tends to run in families that have a high incidence of allergic conditions such as asthma and eczema, but many people seem to grow out of the problem as they get older.

 See also **Conjunctivitis**, p.58; **Blocked or runny nose**, p.77; **Wheezing**, p.103.

What you can do yourself

Most people are able to control their symptoms using over-the-counter remedies. Try the following to see what works best for you.

 • Take an antihistamine to relieve most hay fever symptoms (*see* DRUG REMEDIES, right).

 • Cromolyn sodium nasal spray (*see* DRUG REMEDIES, right) can be used to prevent or relieve a runny nose.

 • For temporary relief of itchy, red eyes, use antihistamine/decongestant eyedrops (*see* DRUG REMEDIES, right).

 • Decongestant sprays can be used in the short term to clear a blocked nose (*see* DRUG REMEDIES, right). They can also be used to help clear your nose before you start a course of cromolyn sodium nasal spray, allowing the spray to work more effectively.

 • Avoid substances that can further irritate your nose and eyes, such as tobacco smoke or dust, perfumes, or strong-smelling chemicals.

• When the pollen count is high (usually on hot, dry, windy days at midmorning and early evening), stay indoors as much as possible, keeping windows and doors closed. In a car, keep windows and air vents closed. Some newer cars have pollen filters.

• Dry clothes inside if possible. If you do dry laundry outside, bring it in before the evening.

• Take a shower and wash your hair before bed to remove pollen that has built up during the day.

DRUG REMEDIES

Antihistamine pills (*see* p.178) are a convenient treatment that can be used as a one-time treatment or regularly. They quickly relieve most hay fever symptoms, including sneezing.

Cromolyn sodium nasal spray (*see* p.181) helps relieve a runny nose. If you know you are prone to hay fever, start using the nasal spray a week or two before the start of the hay fever season. It needs to be used continuously.

Antihistamine/decongestant eyedrops (*see* p.178) contain the antihistamine pheniramine and the decongestant naphazalone. They act quickly to provide temporary relief of itchy, red, and watery eyes associated with hay fever.

Decongestants (*see* p.181), available as nasal sprays, act quickly. They are effective when used occasionally to provide temporary relief from symptoms. Do not use them for more than 7 days, however, or they may make you feel more congested when you stop.

 ## Seek medical advice

Arrange to see your doctor if:

• There is no improvement after you have been using home treatments for 2–3 weeks

Sore throat

Sore throats are very common. In addition to a painful throat, you may have difficulty swallowing, a mild cough, hoarse voice, fever, headache, and enlarged glands in the front of your neck. Normally, the soreness gets worse over a period of 2–3 days, then begins to clear up. A sore throat is usually caused by a viral infection, and often develops with a cold or the flu. It may also be a symptom of mononucleosis. Another possible cause is tonsillitis – an infection of the tonsils at the back of the throat. If you have tonsillitis, you are likely to feel even more feverish and generally ill. Your tonsils will be enlarged and may have pus on them, and your throat will feel uncomfortable when you try to eat or drink.

What you can do yourself

Use these home treatments to make your throat feel more comfortable while you get better.

- Drink at least 8 glasses of fluids a day, even if this feels painful, because your throat will feel worse if it is dry and/or if you become dehydrated. Warm drinks with honey and lemon are particularly soothing (*see* NATURAL REMEDIES, p.30). Avoid undiluted citrus juices because they are acidic and may irritate your throat.

- Try a throat treatment: suck a lozenge or use a spray containing a local anesthetic to numb your throat (*see* DRUG REMEDIES, right).

- Have bland, soft foods, such as rice pudding and yogurt, while your throat is sore. Ice cream is cooling and soothing. It will also help encourage a child with a sore throat to eat.

- Take an analgesic or try a pain-relieving gargle (*see* DRUG REMEDIES, right).

- You can also gargle with a salt solution. Dissolve half a teaspoon of salt in a glass of warm water, gargle for 30 seconds, then spit it out.

- Don't use mouthwashes containing alcohol because they will dry your mouth and tongue.

- Rest your voice. Avoid talking too much or straining your voice.

- Keep your rooms humidified to keep your throat moist. Put a bowl of water in a room, hang a wet towel close to a radiator, or use a humidifier.

- Avoid spending time in smoky or polluted environments because this will make your symptoms worse. If you smoke, try to stop or at least cut down while you have a sore throat.

DRUG REMEDIES

Mouth and throat treatments (*see* p.187) containing local anesthetics will numb a sore throat temporarily and make it easier for you to drink and eat.

Analgesics Take acetaminophen (*see* p.177) or ibuprofen (*see* p.185). You can give a child acetaminophen drops, liquid medicine, or chewable pills. Adults can also gargle with 1 or 2 soluble aspirin (*see* p.179) dissolved in water; repeat 3–4 times a day as needed.

CAUTION: Children and teenagers should not use aspirin before a doctor is consulted about Reye's syndrome, a rare but serious illness.

Pain relief
Tilt your head back and gargle with the solution, or rinse for 1–2 minutes before spitting it out.

✚ Seek medical advice

Arrange to see your doctor if:

- A sore throat becomes more severe or has not got better after 5 days
- You are finding it very difficult to swallow
- You develop other symptoms, such as joint pains or swellings in your armpits or groin

Hoarseness and loss of voice

When your voice sounds scratchy or husky and you have difficulty making yourself heard, the cause is usually inflammation of the voice box (laryngitis) due to an infection such as a cold. Your throat may be sore as well or feel as if there is a lump in it. You can also suddenly lose your voice as a result of overuse – for example, after shouting at a football game. When hoarseness develops gradually, it is usually because of prolonged overuse of the voice, smoking, or reflux of stomach acid (heartburn) irritating the voice box. In rare cases, a hoarse voice is a symptom of cancer of the larynx.

See also Sore throat, p.81; Heartburn, p.107.

What you can do yourself

Hoarseness and loss of voice are usually temporary, lasting for no more than a week. The following measures will help you recover your voice.

- Rest your voice as much as possible. Don't talk or whisper. Whispering can strain your vocal cords even more than normal speech.

- Drink plenty of warm fluids to soothe your throat and 6–8 glasses of water a day to keep it lubricated. Don't drink caffeinated drinks or alcohol.

- Eat soft foods that can be swallowed easily.

- Avoid dry or smoky environments, which can dry the throat and aggravate hoarseness.

 - If your throat feels sore, take an analgesic (*see* DRUG REMEDIES, right).

- Try a steam inhalation to soothe inflammation and loosen secretions (*see* PRACTICAL TECHNIQUE: STEAM INHALATION, p.79).

- Don't gargle – it does not help, and the alcohol in some gargles may cause more irritation. Cough medicines won't relieve hoarseness, either.

Seek medical advice

Arrange to see your doctor promptly if:

- Your throat is still hoarse after 2 weeks in spite of following the advice given above
- You are also having difficulty breathing or swallowing

DRUG REMEDIES

Analgesics, such as acetaminophen (*see* p.177), will help to relieve the discomfort if your throat is painful as well as hoarse.

PREVENTION

Protecting your throat If you are prone to hoarseness and losing your voice, try using the following measures to help prevent recurrences.

- Drink 6–8 glasses of water a day. Keep a bottle of water on your desk at work, and take frequent sips.
- If your work involves speaking to a group or class, try to avoid raising or straining your voice. Organize smaller groups and sit closer together. If you need to address a large audience, ask for a microphone.
- Shouting or screaming puts unnecessary strain on your voice, so try to control anger or anxiety if it makes you prone to doing this.
- Stop smoking and avoid spending long periods of time in smoky atmospheres.
- Try not to cough or clear your throat forcibly.
- Try to breathe through your nose. Breathing through your mouth dries the lining of your throat and introduces cold, unfiltered air into the lungs, which contributes to hoarseness.
- Use a humidifier in your home, or place bowls of water beside a radiator, to keep the air moist.

Nosebleed

Nosebleeds are common in children, but some adults have them occasionally, too. Common causes include nose picking and forceful nose blowing, but nosebleeds often occur for no obvious reason. Your nose is more likely to bleed if its delicate lining is irritated because of a cold or an allergy, or if it becomes dry and cracked due to a dry atmosphere. Although most nosebleeds are little more than a temporary nuisance, bleeding is sometimes a symptom of an underlying illness.

WARNING

Seek immediate medical help if:
- Bleeding is very severe
- You have hit your head or neck
- You are vomiting swallowed blood
- You are taking aspirin or any blood-thinning medication

What you can do yourself

Nosebleeds may look alarming but can usually be stopped fairly easily and prevented from restarting. In older people, a nosebleed can be more difficult to control. Try the following measures.

Controlling a nosebleed
- Stay calm. If you are helping someone else with a nosebleed, be reassuring.

- Take steps to stop the bleeding (*see* PRACTICAL TECHNIQUE, right).

- Don't push tissues or cotton balls into your nostrils to try to stop the bleeding.

Once bleeding has stopped
- Try not to blow your nose for 24 hours afterward. Make sure that you don't pick your nose.

- If you feel the need to sneeze, do so with your mouth open.

- Avoid drinking hot liquids or alcohol, or smoking.

- Sleep with your head raised on 2 or 3 pillows.

- Avoid vigorous exercise for 24 hours after a nosebleed has occurred.

- In dry, heated rooms, use a humidifier or place a bowl of water close to a radiator.

- If you are prone to nosebleeds because your nose tends to be dry and crusted inside, rub petroleum jelly inside your nostrils a few times a day to soften and protect the delicate membrane that lines the nose. Alternatively, use saline nose drops to keep the nasal membrane moist (*see* DRUG REMEDIES, right).

PRACTICAL TECHNIQUE

Stopping a nosebleed These steps should stop a nosebleed within 5–10 minutes.
- Lean forward slightly. If you are feeling faint, sit down and lean forward.
- Firmly pinch the soft part of your nose for 5–10 minutes. Breathe through your mouth.
- If bleeding persists after 10 minutes, pinch for another 5–10 minutes. If this does not work, seek immediate medical help.

Pinching your nose
Pinch the soft part just below the bridge.

DRUG REMEDIES

Saline nose drops (*see* p.188) are available from your pharmacist and are safe to use on children. If the lining of your nose is dry, use them several times a day.

Seek medical advice

Arrange to see your doctor if:
- You are getting recurrent nosebleeds
- You are feeling generally unwell
- You are bruising easily

Snoring

Snoring is the sound of the soft palate (the back of the roof of the mouth) vibrating when it relaxes during sleep. Although it does no harm in itself, it can disturb the snorer and anyone who shares the same bed or room. Snoring can be provoked by conditions that cause swelling in the nasal and throat passages, such as hay fever, colds, and throat or sinus infections, as well as combinations of lifestyle factors such as drinking alcohol, being overweight, and smoking. More men than women snore, and the tendency to do so increases from middle age onward. In children, it is often due to enlarged tonsils and adenoids.

 ## See your doctor first

Make an appointment to see your doctor if you or your partner notice the following symptom in addition to snoring:

● You have pauses in breathing of 10 seconds or more during sleep. (You may wake suddenly as you take a deep breath to compensate.)

What you can do yourself

In addition to being embarrassing, snoring can be disruptive to relationships. Try some of the following measures to get a better night's sleep.

● You are more likely to snore when sleeping on your back. Train yourself to sleep on your side by tucking a pillow into your back or sewing a tennis ball into the back of your nightclothes.

● Lose any excess weight; this will reduce fat deposits around the back of your mouth and nose.

● Reduce your alcohol intake and avoid drinking any alcohol in the 4–5 hours before you go to bed.

● Give up smoking, since tobacco smoke irritates the linings of the nose and throat.

● Don't use sleeping pills or sedative antihistamines because they relax the soft palate.

● Try self-help measures to relieve any nasal congestion (*see* BLOCKED OR RUNNY NOSE, p.77).

 ● Use an adhesive strip that keeps the nasal passages open (*see* PRACTICAL TECHNIQUE, right).

● If your partner's snoring is making it impossible for you to sleep, try gently nudging or calling to your partner so that he or she changes position but does not wake up.

PRACTICAL TECHNIQUE

Using a nasal strip One remedy for snoring uses an adhesive strip attached to the nose to make breathing easier. Stick the strip across the soft part of your nose before you go to bed. The adhesive pad has bands of plastic embedded in it that tighten and lift the sides of the nose, helping maintain airflow while you sleep.

Applying the strip
The strip should be attached to the soft part of your nose, just above the nostrils.

 ## Seek further medical advice

Arrange to see your doctor if:

● The snoring is not helped by the measures on this page and is disrupting your sleep and/or your partner's sleep
● You feel tired and irritable during the day

HEAD, BACK, AND LIMB PROBLEMS

Headache

The most common type of headache is a tension headache. You may feel pressure around your head and behind your eyes and have a stiff neck and shoulder muscles. Tension headaches usually last for a few hours and are commonly due to stress, fatigue, or poor posture, which may cause tension in the neck and scalp. Other triggers include certain foods, poor eyesight, hunger or dehydration, and changes in the menstrual cycle. Headaches also occur with illnesses such as the flu and can be a symptom of meningitis.

 See also **Migraine**, p.86.

> ### WARNING
> Seek urgent medical attention if the pain is sudden and incapacitating, follows head injury, or occurs with:
> - Drowsiness and blurred vision
> - Stiff neck; sensitivity to light; fever; vomiting; possibly a rash (*see* p.150)
> - Limb weakness

What you can do yourself

Use the following measures at the first sign of a headache to stop it from becoming worse.

- Take an analgesic (*see* DRUG REMEDIES, right). It is best to start taking it as soon as the headache begins, before the pain becomes intense.

- Take a hot bath or shower to help your neck and shoulder muscles relax.

- Try using heat to soothe the pain: fill a hot-water bottle, wrap it in a towel, and rest your head on it.

- Ask a partner or friend to massage the muscles at the back of your neck, using his or her fingertips in a gentle circular motion.

- Rest in a quiet room, in darkness or with dimmed lights. Make sure you get enough sleep at night.

- If headaches are linked to stress, try aerobic exercise (such as brisk walking), yoga, or practice deep breathing and muscle relaxation exercises (*see* PRACTICAL TECHNIQUES, pp.20–21).

- Have your eyesight checked.

- If you work at a desk or computer workstation, get up and walk around regularly to reduce tension in your neck and shoulders.

- Avoid drinking alcohol and caffeine in excess, and smoking, all of which can lead to headaches.

DRUG REMEDIES

Analgesics Take ibuprofen (*see* p.185) or acetaminophen (*see* p.177) for a headache, but don't use analgesics for more than a few days at a time. If you take them regularly your body will become accustomed to them and you may have continuing headaches as each dose of medication wears off.

Choosing analgesics
Soluble analgesics and liquid capsules are absorbed fast. Chewable tablets dissolve in the mouth.

 ## Seek medical advice

Arrange to see your doctor if:

- The headache has not cleared up within a day or two or is becoming more severe
- You feel that your headache is not a simple tension headache
- You have recurrent headaches or need to use analgesics regularly

Migraine

A migraine is an intense, throbbing headache, usually on one side of your head and often behind one eye or temple. You may feel nauseated or vomit, and be particularly sensitive to bright light and loud noises. A migraine can last for anything from a few hours to 3 days and may be so debilitating that it prevents normal activities. Shortly before an attack, some people have warning symptoms (known as aura), such as visual disturbances and an altered sense of taste and smell. Factors that can trigger migraines in susceptible people include stress; changes in sleep routine; certain foods and drinks; and, in women, fluctuating hormone levels.

 ## See your doctor first

See your doctor to confirm that your symptoms are due to a migraine.

What you can do yourself

Use the following treatments and self-help measures as soon as an attack begins.

- Take an analgesic at the first sign of an attack. If you feel sick or are vomiting, take a migraine remedy (see DRUG REMEDIES, right).

- If possible, lie down in a dark, quiet room with pillows to support your head. Try to sleep.

- Sip water throughout the day, especially if you have been vomiting.

- Wear sunglasses if you are out in bright daylight.

PREVENTION

Reducing attacks To reduce the frequency and severity of migraine attacks, try these measures.

- Keep a journal for a few weeks, noting when you have migraines and any possible contributory factors. Foods such as red wine, chocolate, and cheese are common triggers. Too much caffeine or cutting back suddenly on your regular intake can cause migraine.
- If stress is a factor, try to reduce it (see pp.20–21).
- Eat regularly and drink 6–8 glasses of water a day.
- Keep to a regular sleep pattern. Too little or too much sleep can trigger a migraine.
 - Taking the herb feverfew may help to prevent migraine attacks (see NATURAL REMEDIES, right).

DRUG REMEDIES

Analgesics, such as acetaminophen (see p.177), aspirin (see p.179), or ibuprofen (see p.185), should be taken as soon as symptoms or aura begin to develop. CAUTION: Children and tennagers should not use aspirin before a doctor is consulted about Reye's syndrome, a rare but serious illness.

Migraine remedies (see p.186) combine analgesics and caffeine (which enhances the analgesic effect) in one pill to help relieve the headache, nausea, and sensitivity to light and sound associated with a migraine.

NATURAL REMEDIES

Feverfew (see p.182) is a garden herb that is available as supplements. Some people find that it reduces the frequency of migraine attacks.

Feverfew capsules
Try taking the capsules for a few weeks to see if they help.

 ## Seek further medical advice

Arrange to see your doctor if:

- Your migraines are not getting better with self-help or prescribed treatments
- You are having frequent or severe attacks

Sore or stiff neck

A painful or stiff neck is usually due to a muscle strain or spasm, caused by poor posture or a minor injury. You may suffer from a stiff neck and shoulders if you sit hunched over a computer for long periods, or you may wake with a stiff neck if you sleep awkwardly. Pain may also be felt in your head, shoulders, arms, or upper back and may be worse when you turn your head or look up or down. Pain and stiffness can also be due to a "whiplash injury," arthritis in the spine, or an underlying illness or injury.

WARNING

Seek immediate medical help if:
- You have a sore or stiff neck with any or all of the following symptoms: fever, vomiting, headache, dislike of bright light, and a rash (*see* p.150)

 ## See your doctor first

Make an appointment to see your doctor if:

- You have a sore or stiff neck after an injury
- You have tingling, numbness, or weakness in an arm or hand; weight loss; or fever

What you can do yourself

A stiff and sore neck due to muscle strain or poor posture should begin to ease within 2–3 days using these home treatments.

- Continue with normal activities as far as the pain allows. If the pain is bad, however, you may need to rest your neck for the first day or two.

- A padded collar may help support your neck. You can make a collar by rolling up a hand towel and putting it into one leg of a pair of pantyhose, then gently securing it around your neck. Only wear a collar for a short period, and don't wear it at night.

- Start gentle neck exercises as soon as you are able to do so (*see* PRACTICAL TECHNIQUE, right).

- Take an analgesic (*see* DRUG REMEDIES, right).

- To relieve a muscle spasm, stand under a warm shower, or place a covered hot-water bottle or a heating pad on the back of your neck, for 15 minutes every few hours.

- Use a supportive pillow in bed. Alternatively, make a neck-support pillow by tying a scarf or bandage around the middle of a pillow to form a butterfly shape. Rest your head on the narrow part.

PRACTICAL TECHNIQUE

Neck exercise The following exercise will help loosen a stiff neck.

- Stand straight, or sit on the edge of a chair looking straight ahead. Drop your head to one side, toward your shoulder. Keep your shoulder down.
- Hold for a few seconds, then raise your head again. Repeat on the other side.
- Repeat the exercise 5 times on each side, about 3 times a day. Exercise to the point of discomfort, but don't try to exercise through pain.
- Gradually increase the range of movement. Stop at once, however, if the pain gets worse or if it begins to move into your arm or hand.

DRUG REMEDIES

Analgesics will help relieve the discomfort of a stiff or sore neck and will help you keep your neck mobile. Take acetaminophen (*see* p.177), or ibuprofen (*see* p.185), which may be more effective.

 ## Seek further medical advice

Arrange to see your doctor if:

- The soreness or stiffness is getting worse
- The problem has not eased after 2 days

Lower back pain

Most sudden back pain is due to a sprain or a small tear in a muscle or ligament. You may have a nagging ache in your lower back or a sharp, localized pain and stiffness due to a muscle spasm in the area. Sciatica is pain that travels through one buttock to the leg and foot, sometimes with numbness, tingling, and weakness in the leg. It is caused by trapping or irritation of the sciatic nerve, often due to a "slipped disk" between the bones of the spine. The usual causes of back pain and sciatica include lifting awkwardly or sudden twisting, but factors such as poor posture, pregnancy, and being inactive or unfit may make the back more vulnerable.

WARNING

Seek immediate medical help if:
- You have difficulty controlling your bowels or bladder; tingling and/or numbness in the anal or genital area; or muscle weakness
- Back pain follows an injury

See your doctor first

Make an appointment to see your doctor if:

- You have symptoms of sciatica
- Back pain has been developing slowly and is gradually getting worse
- You are losing weight or have a fever

What you can do yourself

An episode of back pain usually gets better within a few weeks. Take these steps to ease pain, staying as active as possible rather than resting in bed.

- If the pain is tolerable, try to continue normal activities as much as possible. Gradually increase what you do each day, but don't overdo things. Stop any activity that makes the pain worse.

- If the pain is so severe that you cannot move, rest in bed for a day or two. As soon as you feel able to do so, get out of bed and start moving, even if it causes some discomfort.

- Your mattress needs to be firm, but not too hard. If you have an old, sagging mattress that does not support your back, put a board under it. You will probably find that lying on your side is more comfortable than lying on your back.

 - While your back is painful, try to move in ways that are less likely to bring on or worsen the pain (*see* PRACTICAL TECHNIQUE, right).

 - Take analgesics to relieve pain and stiffness (*see* DRUG REMEDIES, opposite page).

PRACTICAL TECHNIQUE

Moving without pain Getting out of bed awkwardly can cause sudden, painful twinges when you have back pain. This sequence of movements will get you on your feet with minimum strain on your spine, so continue to use them even when your back is no longer painful.

1 *Lying flat on your back, bring your knees up to hip level and roll yourself slowly onto your side, facing the edge of the bed.*

2 *Swing your legs to the edge of the bed and lower your feet to the floor. Use your arms to push yourself into a sitting position.*

3 *Using your arms and your leg muscles to push yourself up, slowly rise to a standing position. Reverse the procedure when you get back into bed.*

What you can do yourself *continued...*

 ● Rubbing the sore area with a counterirritant cream or gel may help soothe the pain for a short while (*see* DRUG REMEDIES, right).

 ● Holding a wrapped hot-water bottle or heating pad against your back may help relieve pain, particularly if there is muscle spasm. You can also direct warm water onto the small of your back when in the shower.

✚ Seek further medical advice

Arrange to see your doctor if:

● The back pain is getting worse or is not easing within 48 hours
● You develop any of the symptoms listed in the Warning box

PREVENTION

Avoiding back pain If you are prone to back pain, you may be able to prevent further episodes by taking particular care of your back.

● Wear comfortable shoes with a low heel.
● If you are overweight, lose weight – it will help take pressure off your back.
● Walking, swimming, or a course of Pilates or yoga exercises will help strengthen your back muscles. Your doctor or physical therapist can also recommend back-strengthening exercises.
 ● Try to improve your posture when you walk, stand, and sit, both while you have back pain and afterward (*see* PRACTICAL TECHNIQUE, right). You should also practice safe ways of lifting and moving heavy objects to reduce the risk of straining your back (*see* PREVENTION: LIFTING HEAVY OBJECTS, p.112).

DRUG REMEDIES

Analgesics include acetaminophen (*see* p.177) and ibuprofen (*see* p.185). Ibuprofen also has an anti-inflammatory effect, which will reduce stiffness in your back, making it easier for you to try some gentle movement.

Counterirritants (*see* p.181), available as creams, gels, or sprays, produce a tingling sensation in the skin that soothes pain temporarily. Some warm the area; others have a cooling effect.

PRACTICAL TECHNIQUES

Standing and walking When you are standing or walking, pull your shoulders slightly back and down, holding your trunk straight. Try to balance your weight evenly over both feet.

Driving Angle the driver's seat backward very slightly and position it so you can reach the hand and foot controls easily. While you are driving, check from time to time that your arms are relaxed and your shoulders are not hunched.

Sitting Sit with your back straight, your bottom pushed into the back of a chair, and your feet flat on the floor. Choose a chair that is the right height to allow you to do this, with an upright back that supports the small of your back. The seat should support the full length of your thighs but should not put too much pressure on the backs of your thighs. When using a computer, the top of the screen should be at eye level. Your arms and thighs should be parallel to the floor and your keyboard and mouse should be close enough to your body that you don't have to stretch to use them.

Good posture
Sit far back in the chair, with your back straight and your lower back supported by the backrest. Keep both feet flat on the floor.

Shoulder pain

Shoulder pain can be continuous or it may occur only when you make certain movements, such as circling your arm. The pain may also radiate down one arm. The usual cause is inflammation of the muscles and tendons that surround the shoulder joint. This may develop if you strain your shoulder, for example during sports or other strenuous activities. Gradual wear and tear on the joint from osteoarthritis can also cause shoulder pain.

> ## WARNING
> Seek immediate medical help if shoulder pain is associated with:
> - Pain or heaviness in your chest
> - Sweating
> - Breathlessness

 ## See your doctor first

Make an appointment to see your doctor if you have shoulder pain after a fall or injury.

What you can do yourself

There are several things you can do to reduce pain and stiffness and get your shoulder moving normally.

- Take an analgesic to relieve the pain (*see* DRUG REMEDIES, right).

- Apply an ice pack (such as a bag of frozen peas or crushed ice, wrapped in a wet towel). Hold for 10 minutes. Reapply 2–3 times a day for the first 2 days.

- Massaging a counterirritant cream or gel into the sore area may help soothe the pain for a short while (*see* DRUG REMEDIES, right).

- Rest the shoulder for a few days, but try to keep it mobile by gently shrugging from time to time. If you don't, it may get persistently stiff and painful ("frozen shoulder"). As the pain eases, start exercising your shoulder (*see* PRACTICAL TECHNIQUE, right).

- At night, lie on the pain-free side and cuddle a cushion with the other arm for support. If you lie on your back, support your arm with a pillow.

- Make sure you keep your armpit on the affected side clean and dry to avoid soreness.

 ## Seek further medical advice

Arrange to see your doctor if:
- Your shoulder is becoming more painful
- It is not getting better after 2–3 days

DRUG REMEDIES

Analgesics Take acetaminophen (*see* p.177) or ibuprofen (*see* p.185) to relieve pain. Ibuprofen has an anti-inflammatory effect, which will help reduce any swelling and stiffness.

Counterirritants (*see* p.181) are creams and gels that produce a tingling sensation in the skin, which soothes pain temporarily. Some products have a warming effect and increase blood flow to the area; others have a cooling effect.

PRACTICAL TECHNIQUE

Shoulder exercises Do these exercises twice a day to improve flexibility. You may find it helpful to do them under a warm shower. Gradually increase the range of movement as the pain lessens.

1 *Put your arms out to the side and lift them, stopping as soon as it becomes uncomfortable. Slowly drop them to your sides. Repeat 5 times.*

2 *Put your arms out to the front and lift them until you start to feel discomfort. Slowly drop them to your sides. Repeat 5 times.*

Tennis or golfer's elbow

Also called tendinitis, tennis or golfer's elbow is inflammation of the tendons where they attach to the bone at the elbow. The main symptom is pain in the forearm that becomes worse when you try to pick up objects, shake hands, or use any action that strains the affected tendon. Overuse of your wrist and forearm while playing sports is the usual cause, although inflammation can also occur when you use a screwdriver or similar tool too vigorously. Tennis elbow affects the tendon on the outer side of your elbow, and golfer's elbow involves the tendon on the inner side.

 ## See your doctor first

Make an appointment to see your doctor if:

- You develop pain in your elbow after an injury
- Your elbow is swollen and feels hot

What you can do yourself

There are several ways to reduce elbow pain. It's important to start treatment as soon as possible.

- Rest your arm and hand whenever you can, and reduce activities that put strain on the tendon.

- Apply an ice pack (such as a bag of frozen peas or crushed ice, wrapped in a wet towel) to the painful area. Hold in place for about 10 minutes. Reapply 2–3 times a day for the first 2 days.

- Try wearing an elbow strap, available from your pharmacist, to help ease the pain of tendinitis.

 - Take an analgesic (*see* DRUG REMEDIES, right).

 - Massaging a counterirritant into the sore area may help to soothe pain (*see* DRUG REMEDIES, right).

 - When you are ready to resume playing sports, do elbow-stretching exercises before you play (*see* PRACTICAL TECHNIQUE, right). Ask your doctor or physical therapist for advice on other exercises to strengthen your elbow joint.

 ## Seek further medical advice

Arrange to see your doctor if:

- The pain does not start to subside after 1–2 weeks of the treatment described above

 ### DRUG REMEDIES

Analgesics Take acetaminophen (*see* p.177) or ibuprofen (*see* p.185) to relieve pain. Ibuprofen has an anti-inflammatory effect, which will help reduce any swelling and stiffness.

Counterirritants (*see* p.181) are creams and gels that produce a tingling sensation in the skin, which soothes pain temporarily. Some products have a warming effect and increase blood flow to the area; others have a cooling effect.

 ### PRACTICAL TECHNIQUE

Elbow stretches Doing these exercises will warm you up and help to prevent elbow strains.

1 *Hold your forearms and hands straight out in front of you, with your palms downward. Lightly clench your fists and flex your wrists up and down 10 times.*

2 *Hold your arms and hands straight out in front of you. Keeping your elbows straight, rotate your hands from palms upward to palms downward 10 times.*

Hip pain

The most common cause of pain and stiffness in the hip is wear and tear due to arthritis. This condition usually affects older people; if you have it, you may feel pain in your thigh, buttock, or groin as well as in your hip. Another cause is bursitis, in which the fluid-filled sac that cushions the hip joint becomes inflamed because of overuse or injury. Bursitis causes pain on the outside of the thigh, close to the hip, that gets worse when you climb stairs or lie on the affected side.

WARNING

Seek immediate medical help if:
- You develop hip pain after an accident or fall
- Walking is difficult, or you cannot put weight on the affected leg
- You have a fever with hip pain

See your doctor first

Make an appointment to see your doctor if you have hip pain to establish the cause.

What you can do yourself

If you have an episode of hip pain, try the following measures to help relieve the discomfort.

- Take an analgesic; massaging the hip with a counterirritant can also be soothing (*see* DRUG REMEDIES, right).

- Try to keep moving gently, resting your hip and leg whenever you can. Avoid activity that brings on pain or makes it worse.

- If you have bursitis, try applying an ice pack (such as a bag of frozen peas or crushed ice wrapped in a wet towel). Hold in place for about 10 minutes. Reapply 2–3 times a day for the first 48 hours.

- If you have arthritis, hold a covered hot-water bottle or a heating pad on your hip.

- Sleep on a firm mattress. Try not to lie on the hip.

- For arthritis, try a supplement of glucosamine and/or chondroitin (*see* NATURAL REMEDIES, right).

Seek further medical advice

Arrange to see your doctor if:
- Your hip is not improving after a week, or is getting worse
- You develop pain in other joints

DRUG REMEDIES

Analgesics include acetaminophen (*see* p.177) and ibuprofen (*see* p.185), which also has an anti-inflammatory effect.

Counterirritants (*see* p.181) are creams and gels that produce a tingling sensation, which soothes pain temporarily. Some products have a warming effect; others have a cooling effect.

NATURAL REMEDIES

Glucosamine and chondroitin (*see* p.183) occur naturally in joint cartilage. Taking a supplement of either, or both combined, may reduce pain and stiffness and slow the progress of arthritis.

PREVENTION

Avoiding hip pain Once the pain has subsided, take these steps to help prevent recurrences.

- Lose any excess weight, since it puts extra pressure on your hip.
- Cycle or swim regularly to build the muscles that support your hip joint.

Safe swimming
Avoid doing the breaststroke since it can strain your hip.

Knee pain

As main weight-bearing joints, knees are easily strained or injured; one or both knees may be painful and may be swollen, warm to the touch, and difficult to move. A sudden twisting movement is a common cause of injury, while inflammation in the joint or in the fluid-filled sacs surrounding it (bursitis) and arthritis are longer-term causes of pain and stiffness.

 See also **Sprains and strains**, p.160.

WARNING

Seek immediate medical help if:

- You have severe knee pain and/or your knee is swollen, red, and hot, and you have a fever
- You cannot walk after an injury and/or you cannot move your knee

 ## See your doctor first

Make an appointment to see your doctor if:

- You are concerned about a knee injury
- You have pain in other joints and/or you have had knee pain for some time

What you can do yourself

There are several home treatments that will help relieve pain and increase your mobility.

- If you have injured your knee, use the R.I.C.E. procedure (*see* PRACTICAL TECHNIQUE, p.160).

 - Take an analgesic (*see* DRUG REMEDIES, right).

 - Massaging your knee with a counterirritant cream or gel may also help soothe the pain (*see* DRUG REMEDIES, right).

- To prevent stiffness, move your knee frequently as far as the pain allows. Gradually increase the range of movement as the pain subsides.

 - If your knee pain is due to arthritis, taking a supplement of glucosamine and/or chondroitin may help in the long term (*see* NATURAL REMEDIES, right).

- Lose weight if you need to do so, because being overweight puts extra stress on the knee joint.

- Wear comfortable shoes with a well-cushioned sole and a low heel.

- Regular exercise, such as walking up stairs or cycling, will strengthen the leg muscles that help to protect and support your joints.

 ### DRUG REMEDIES

Analgesics include acetaminophen (*see* p.177) and ibuprofen (*see* p.185), which also has an anti-inflammatory effect.

Counterirritants (*see* p.181) are creams and gels that produce a tingling sensation, which soothes pain temporarily. Some products have a warming effect; others have a cooling effect.

 ### NATURAL REMEDIES

Glucosamine and chondroitin (*see* p.183) are naturally occurring substances found in joint cartilage. Taking supplements of either, or a combination of both, may relieve pain and stiffness and slow the progress of arthritis.

Arthritis relief
It may take at least a month for glucosamine and/or chondroitin supplements to have an effect.

 ## Seek further medical advice

Arrange to see your doctor if:

- Pain and swelling from an injury are not subsiding after about 2 days
- The pain is becoming worse
- You develop new symptoms

Leg cramps

A cramp is a painful spasm, usually in one or more calf or foot muscles. The muscle becomes hard and knotted, and hurts if you try to move it. The pain usually lasts for only a few minutes. You may get a cramp on waking up or after sitting or lying awkwardly. If you get it during exercise or strenuous work, it is usually due to overusing muscles, heat, dehydration, or salt and mineral loss. Swimmers can get cramps if they become cold and exhausted.

WARNING

Seek urgent medical help if:
- You have continuous pain deep in your calf or in a leg vein
- Your leg is hot, red, or swollen; turns blue or white; or feels cold

What you can do yourself

Although a cramp will subside on its own, the steps below will help minimize discomfort.

- If you get cramps during exercise, stop. Gently massage the muscle. If the spasm is in your calf, stretch it. Pull your toes toward your knee, letting your ankle bend. Hold until the muscle relaxes.

- If the cramp occurs while you are in bed, get up and wiggle your foot or walk around. If it persists, try stretching the muscle as above.

- Try heat, particularly for cramps due to swimming. Take a warm bath or shower, then wrap a warm towel around the muscle. Put on warm clothing or cover your leg with a blanket afterward. However, for cramps caused by overuse, try an ice pack. Wrap a bag of frozen peas or crushed ice in a wet towel, and hold it on the muscle for 10 minutes.

PREVENTION

Avoiding cramps If you are prone to cramps, the following tips may help prevent attacks.

- Drink 8 glasses of water a day. Have 1–2 glasses 2 hours before any exercise; $\frac{1}{2}$–1 glass every 15–20 minutes during exercise; and plenty of fluids afterward.
- Warm up thoroughly before you exercise, and ease off gradually afterward. Stop when you need to rest.
- Do calf-stretching exercises to relieve and prevent cramps (*see* PRACTICAL TECHNIQUE, right).
- Eat foods rich in potassium, magnesium, and calcium, such as avocados, bananas, oranges, milk, dark-leaved vegetables, whole-grain foods, and nuts.
- Stop smoking; it contributes to the risk of cramps.

PRACTICAL TECHNIQUE

Calf-stretching exercise Try this exercise to relieve cramps and as a daily routine to prevent further episodes. Do it before and after using your leg muscles for long periods and before going to bed if you are prone to leg cramps at night.

1 *Stand about an arm's length from a wall with one leg in front of the other and your hands flat against the wall at shoulder height.*

2 *Keeping your feet flat on the floor, lean forward, bending the front knee and pressing the rear heel into the ground. You will feel the calf muscle of the rear leg stretch. Repeat the exercise with the other leg.*

Press the back heel into the ground

Bend the front knee forward

Seek medical advice

Arrange to see your doctor if:

- Cramps are not relieved by these measures, or they become more severe or frequent

Varicose veins

Varicose veins are bluish, distorted veins that bulge beneath the skin, usually on the inside leg, at the back of the calf, or at the ankle. An affected leg may feel heavy, your ankle may swell, and the skin over the veins may be dry and itchy. The problem is more common in women and often runs in families. Pregnancy, constipation, being overweight, or having to stand for long periods increases the risk.

 See also **Swollen ankles**, p.96; **Constipation**, p.115.

Varicose vein on the ankle and foot

What you can do yourself

Although self-help treatments will not get rid of your varicose veins, they will help ease the discomfort and stop the veins from getting worse by improving circulation and muscle tone.

- Try to avoid standing for long periods. When this is unavoidable, flex your calf muscles every few minutes and wiggle your toes. If you sit for long periods, get up every 30 minutes and walk around.

- Don't cross your legs when you sit down, because it restricts blood flow in the lower legs.

- When you relax in an armchair, keep your legs raised on a stool or pile of books, but be careful not to place anything directly under your knees.

- Wear low-heeled or flat shoes; they make your calf muscles work harder when you walk.

- Don't wear girdles, control-top underwear, or pantyhose that constrict your waist or groin and restrict blood flow at the top of your legs. Avoid socks or knee-highs with tight elastic.

- Support stockings may help, especially if you will be standing all day. Put them on first thing in the morning, before your ankles start to swell.

 - Use a moisturizing cream if your skin is dry and itchy over the veins (*see* DRUG REMEDIES, right).

- Take care not to knock the fragile skin over a varicose vein, because this may burst the vein and cause severe bleeding.

- Stop smoking; it can contribute to the risk of varicose veins developing.

DRUG REMEDIES

Moisturizers (*see* p.187), such as water-based cream, can be lightly rubbed into the skin over varicose veins to relieve dryness and itching.

PREVENTION

A few lifestyle changes can help reduce the risk of varicose veins or may help prevent them from getting any worse.

- Lose weight if you are overweight. This will help relieve the pressure on existing veins and may prevent new varicose veins developing.
- Get regular exercise, such as walking, cycling, and swimming, to boost your circulation.
- To prevent constipation, drink 6–8 glasses of water a day. Include plenty of high-fiber food in your diet such as whole-wheat bread; whole-grain cereals; brown rice; vegetables, such as baked potatoes and baked beans; and fresh fruit.
- Wear support stockings or pantyhose regularly if you are pregnant or if your work involves standing for long periods of time.

 ## Seek medical advice

Arrange to see your doctor if:

- **Your varicose veins are getting worse or new ones develop**
- **A vein becomes red and feels warm**
- **The skin over a varicose vein becomes discolored, sore, or weepy**

Swollen ankles

You may develop swollen ankles after a period of inactivity, such as a long car trip or flight, or if you have to spend long periods of time standing up, especially in a hot environment. The swelling is usually caused by a buildup of fluid, as a result of sluggish blood circulation. Your ankles are unlikely to be painful, but you may have an uncomfortable, tight feeling in the skin. The problem can occur with varicose veins, and some women are prone to swollen ankles during pregnancy. Some drugs can contribute to swelling of the ankles, and the problem is sometimes an indication of a heart, kidney, or liver condition.

 See also Varicose veins, p.95.

 ## See your doctor first

Make an appointment to see your doctor if:

- You have pain or tenderness in your calf
- One leg is swollen, with no obvious cause
- You are taking a prescribed medicine that may be causing the problem

What you can do yourself

Try the following measures to reduce swollen ankles or prevent a buildup of fluid.

- To relieve swollen ankles, lie down and prop your legs up 6–12 in (15–30 cm) above the level of your heart. Don't place anything under your knees.

- If you have to stand for long periods, flex your calves every few minutes and wiggle your toes.

- If you are prone to swollen ankles, wear support stockings or tights. Put them on first thing in the morning, before your legs start to swell.

- During long car journeys, stop frequently so that you can stretch your legs.

 - On a long flight, exercise your legs (*see* PRACTICAL TECHNIQUE, right). Try wearing flight socks that use light compression to aid blood flow in the legs.

- Drink 6–8 glasses of water a day to prevent dehydration. Your body will excrete any excess.

- Wear low-heeled or flat shoes; they make the calf muscles work harder than high heels, which improves circulation in the legs.

- Avoid girdles, control-top underwear or pantyhose, and tight socks or knee-highs.

PRACTICAL TECHNIQUE

In-flight exercises During a long flight, do these exercises every 30 minutes to boost blood flow. They will also help prevent the serious disorder deep vein thrombosis ("economy class syndrome"), in which a blood clot develops in the leg.

1 *Starting with your feet flat, keep your heels on the floor and lift your toes as high as you can.*

2 *Now lift your heels high, pressing the balls of your feet into the floor. Do these foot pumps for 30 seconds.*

3 *Stretch one leg out in front of you and circle your foot 8 times in each direction. Change legs and circle the other foot.*

 ## Seek further medical advice

Arrange to see your doctor if:

- Ankle swelling does not subside using the measures described here

Foot pain

Your feet undergo a great deal of wear and pressure. After prolonged standing or walking, they may be aching and swollen, and overactivity can cause pain in the sole or heel, or muscle or tendon strains. Shoes that chafe or squeeze, or sports shoes that do not support the feet, add to the problem. Morton's neuroma (swelling of a nerve between the toe bones) can cause pain in the ball of the foot. Some conditions affecting the whole body, such as gout, diabetes, and arthritis, can also cause foot pain.

 See also **Corns and calluses**, p.42; **Warts and plantar warts**, p.43; **Ingrown toenail**, p.55; **Bunions**, p.98; **Painful heel**, p.99; **Blisters**, p.155.

 ## See your doctor first

Make an appointment to see your doctor if:

- You have diabetes or poor circulation
- Foot pain is due to an injury

What you can do yourself

There are several simple measures that you can take to minimize or relieve foot pain.

- Wear well-fitting shoes in which you can wiggle your toes easily. Avoid shoes with pointed toes or with heels higher than 2 in (5 cm). Alternate pairs of shoes from day to day to give your feet a break.

- Buy new shoes at the end of the day when your feet are likely to be at their largest. Don't buy shoes that are too tight and expect them to stretch.

 - For sports and similar activities, choose shoes that fit comfortably and are appropriate for your chosen activity (*see* PRACTICAL TIPS, right).

- Wear sneakers to and from work if you have to wear formal shoes at the office.

- For extra support and cushioning, an insole may help. Specialized insoles for sports footwear are available from sports shops.

 - If your feet hurt, take an analgesic (*see* DRUG REMEDIES, right).

 - Soak aching feet in the bath, but not for too long otherwise the skin will become dry. Afterward, apply a moisturizer (*see* DRUG REMEDIES, right).

- If the pain is related to a sporting activity, reduce it or stop until the pain has gone.

 ### PRACTICAL TIPS

Choosing sports shoes Your sports shoes should fit comfortably from the start. If you practice a sport regularly, choose shoes designed for that activity; for example, if you run on hard surfaces, you need shoes that support your instep and cushion your heel. When buying new shoes, take the following steps to ensure that they fit correctly.

- Try on the shoes with appropriate sports socks.
- Check that the shoes grip your heels and leave you room to wiggle your toes. Relace them yourself so that they apply even pressure to the top of your feet.
- Walk or run a few steps to decide whether or not the shoes are comfortable.

 ### DRUG REMEDIES

Analgesics, such as ibuprofen (*see* p.185) or acetaminophen (*see* p.177), will help relieve muscle or joint aches. If the pain does not ease after a few days, stop taking them and arrange to see your doctor.

Moisturizers (*see* p.187) will keep your feet soft and help prevent dry areas from developing. Apply moisturizing cream or lotion just after a bath or shower, while your skin is still moist.

 ## Seek further medical advice

Arrange to see your doctor if:

- You still have foot pain after 2–3 weeks of using the measures suggested here

Bunions

A bunion is a bump at the base of the big toe, caused by a deformity of the joint. If you have bunions, your big toes are pushed inward, and the protruding toe joints may become red, tender, and swollen. You may also get corns and calluses over the joints if your shoes rub. Bunions tend to run in families. Pressure from narrow shoes contributes to the problem, making bunions more common in women.

Bunion on right foot

 See also **Corns and calluses**, p.42.

 ## See your doctor first

Make an appointment to see your doctor if you have diabetes or suffer from poor circulation.

What you can do yourself

You cannot get rid of a bunion with self-help treatments, but they will help to relieve the discomfort and prevent it from getting worse.

- Put a felt bunion pad over the sore area to reduce pressure and friction. An arch support may also relieve pressure, and shaped rubber pads between your toes may help keep your big toe in its proper position. Make sure any padding you use does not put pressure on your toes.

- If you have to stand or walk for long periods, take an analgesic (*see* DRUG REMEDIES, right).

- Wear properly fitting shoes with a wide toe area, avoiding pointed styles and heels higher than 2 in (5 cm). Buy new shoes at the end of the day.

- Try foot exercises to help prevent a bunion from getting worse (*see* PRACTICAL TECHNIQUE, right).

- If a bunion is inflamed, apply an ice pack (such as a bag of frozen peas or crushed ice wrapped in a wet towel) several times a day to reduce the swelling.

 ## Seek further medical advice

Arrange to see your doctor if:

- A bunion becomes inflamed or weepy, or causes continual pain

 ### DRUG REMEDIES

Analgesics can be used when your bunion causes severe discomfort. Take ibuprofen (*see* p.185) or acetaminophen (*see* p.177) to relieve the pain.

 ### PRACTICAL TECHNIQUE

Foot exercises If you have the beginnings of a bunion, try these exercises. They strengthen the foot and may prevent the bunion from getting worse.

1 *Practice picking up a pencil or marble from the floor with your toes. You can do this exercise standing up or sitting down.*

2 *Either standing or sitting, put a small, round, strong glass bottle on the floor and roll each foot in turn over it from toe to heel. Do this 10 times.*

3 *Sitting down, keep your heel on the floor and stretch your toes upward, fanning them out as far as you can. Then lift and circle each foot 6 times.*

Painful heel

A common cause of heel pain is inflammation of the sole of the foot (plantar fasciitis), which causes severe pain when you first put pressure on your heel in the morning or after sitting. The problem can be due to activities such as jogging, and is worst when you go barefoot or wear thin-soled shoes. Another cause of heel pain is inflammation of the Achilles tendon (Achilles tendinitis), due to overuse or misuse during exercise. Symptoms include a dull ache in the back of the heel and stiffness in the tendon.

> ## WARNING
>
> Seek immediate medical help if:
> - You feel a "snap" at the back of your ankle during exercise, have severe pain behind your ankle, and/or cannot walk properly
> - Heel pain follows a foot injury

 ## See your doctor first

Make an appointment to see your doctor if you are unsure about the cause of heel pain.

What you can do yourself

Both plantar fasciitis and Achilles tendinitis may be slow to get better. Use the measures below for a few weeks until you see an improvement.

- Try applying an ice pack (such as a bag of frozen peas or crushed ice wrapped in a wet towel) to your heel. Hold it in place for about 10 minutes. Reapply it 2–3 times a day for the first 48 hours.

- If your painful heel is due to plantar fasciitis, massage it for a few minutes in the mornings after a warm bath or shower.

- Take an analgesic such as ibuprofen (*see* DRUG REMEDIES, right).

- Wear shoes with good arch supports and flexible soles. Well-padded sports shoes, laced firmly, will be the most comfortable. If you've strained your Achilles tendon, put a heel pad or piece of foam in your shoe to take the stress off the tendon and make walking less painful.

- Cut back on activities that put pressure on your heel, such as jogging or playing tennis. Try cycling or swimming instead. If you've strained your Achilles tendon, rest completely until the pain has subsided and then begin gentle calf-stretching exercises (*see* PRACTICAL TECHNIQUE, p.94).

> ## DRUG REMEDIES
>
> **Analgesics**, such as ibuprofen (*see* p.185) or acetaminophen (*see* p.177), reduce the discomfort of a painful heel. If it does not improve after 4–5 days, stop taking the analgesic and see your doctor.

> ## PREVENTION
>
> **Protecting your heels** You can protect your heels from damage during exercise, and reduce pressure on them, using the following measures.
>
> - Warm up before exercising. If your heel starts to hurt, stop; don't try to exercise through the pain.
> - If possible, play sports or run on grass or soft indoor surfaces rather than hard surfaces such as pavement.
> - Buy sports shoes designed for your chosen activity and lace them firmly (*see* PRACTICAL TIPS: CHOOSING SPORTS SHOES, p.97). At other times, wear well-fitting shoes with good arch supports, cushioned soles, and heels no higher than 2 in (5 cm).
> - Practice calf-stretching exercises (*see* PRACTICAL TECHNIQUE, p.94) to increase flexibility and reduce the risk of injury to your tendons.
> - If you are overweight, losing weight will help to take some of the strain off your feet.

 ## Seek further medical advice

Arrange to see your doctor if:

- Your heel pain does not subside within a few weeks or becomes more severe

Cold fingers and toes

It is normal for your fingers and toes to react to cold. Some people, though, feel the cold excessively, even if they just put their hands into a refrigerator or hold a cold drink. Poor circulation and underactivity of the thyroid gland can contribute to cold fingers and toes but a more common cause is Raynaud's, in which tiny blood vessels in the fingers (and sometimes the toes) go into spasm, usually in response to cold. The fingers or toes turn white and cold, then blue. As the blood returns, they turn red and may tingle, throb, or feel numb or painful. Raynaud's can also be caused by working with vibrating tools such as chainsaws, some prescribed drugs, and stress, or it may occur as a symptom of diseases affecting blood vessels or joints.

 ### See your doctor first

Make an appointment to see your doctor if your fingers or toes are exceptionally sensitive to cold, to establish the cause.

What you can do yourself

If your fingers and toes are very sensitive to cold, try these steps to reduce the severity of symptoms.

- Try to avoid handling cold objects. Use mittens or a towel to remove food from a refrigerator or freezer. Use a cup holder for a cold drink.

- Stop smoking: nicotine causes narrowing of the blood vessels and contributes to Raynaud's.

- Cut down on caffeinated drinks such as coffee.

 - Keeping your body warm helps the circulation to your hands and feet. Dress warmly when you go out in cold weather (*see* PRACTICAL TIPS, right).

- If your fingers turn white and numb, swing your arms in large circles, clenching and unclenching your hands. Wiggle your toes to increase blood flow. Use hot-air dryers in bathrooms to warm your hands, or soak fingers and toes in warm water.

- Make sure your bedding is warm. An electric blanket may help, as will wearing socks in bed.

 ### Seek further medical advice

Arrange to see your doctor if:

- Your symptoms are persistent or getting worse
- You develop any new, unexplained symptoms, such as joint pains

PRACTICAL TIPS

Dressing to stay warm Put on several thin layers of clothing to trap heat next to your skin; thermal underwear may help.

- Wear a hat and warm your hands before putting on gloves (or mittens, which are even warmer). Try battery-heated gloves or hand heating aids.
- Wear warm socks and put padding in your shoes or boots. Avoid tight-fitting footwear and clothes because they restrict blood circulation.

Heated gloves
These gloves are useful if you have to be outside for long periods of time in cold weather. They are powered by a battery in a pouch in the wrist and stay warm for 5–6 hours.

PREVENTION

Preventing attacks If you regularly have cold fingers and toes, a few lifestyle changes can help prevent or reduce the frequency of attacks.

- Get regular exercise to stimulate the circulation.
- If your problem is triggered by stress, practicing some deep breathing exercises and muscle relaxation techniques (*see* PRACTICAL TECHNIQUES, pp.20–21) may help you reduce it.
- Avoid using vibrating tools if this is a trigger.

CHEST AND ABDOMINAL PROBLEMS

Hiccups

Everyone has an occasional bout of hiccups – short, sharp intakes of air caused by repeated, involuntary spasms of your diaphragm. Although they often occur for no apparent reason, common causes include overeating or eating too fast; eating spicy, very hot, or very cold food; drinking carbonated drinks; or drinking alcohol. Smoking heavily, or emotional factors such as nervousness or shock, can bring on an attack of hiccups, as can a sudden change in temperature. Hiccups usually last for no more than a few minutes. Bouts that last more than a few days can be a sign of illness, and may also lead to difficulty in sleeping and weight loss.

What you can do yourself

Attacks of hiccups disappear of their own accord but if you need to get rid of them quickly, try some of these home remedies.

- Hold your breath for as long as you can, or breathe in and out quickly. Alternatively, breathe into a paper bag (*see* PRACTICAL TECHNIQUE, right).

- Sip iced water, or chew and swallow pieces of crushed ice, for 10–15 minutes.

- Eat a dry piece of bread or a cracker.

- Place a teaspoonful of granulated sugar on the back of your tongue and swallow it.

- Suck on a slice of lemon soaked in Angostura bitters, or sip a small amount of vinegar.

- Pull hard on your tongue, or touch the back of your tongue with your finger or a cotton ball.

- Sit on a chair or on the floor and pull your knees up toward your chest while leaning forward.

- Have someone else startle you unexpectedly. This is sometimes enough to stop a hiccup attack.

 ## Seek medical advice

Arrange to see your doctor if:

- A bout of hiccups has lasted for longer than 24 hours
- You get frequent bouts of hiccups

PRACTICAL TECHNIQUE

Rebreathing Hold a brown paper bag (not a plastic bag) over your nose and mouth, and breathe in and out of it forcefully 10 times. Exhaled air contains higher levels of carbon dioxide than normal, and rebreathing it from a bag may help relax your diaphragm and stop the hiccups.

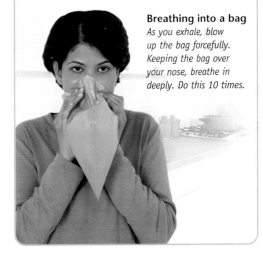

Breathing into a bag
As you exhale, blow up the bag forcefully. Keeping the bag over your nose, breathe in deeply. Do this 10 times.

Coughing

The most common cause of a cough is irritation or inflammation in your lungs or throat due to a cold or flu, a chest infection, or asthma. Irritants such as tobacco smoke, dust, and pollen can make you cough, as can postnasal drip (mucus from the nose dripping down the back of the throat), or regurgitation of stomach acid in heartburn. Some people have a nervous cough that becomes a habit. A cough may be simply dry, tickly, and irritating, or it may bring up mucus (a "productive" cough). Some prescribed drugs cause coughing. Occasionally, however, a cough is a symptom of a serious illness such as cancer.

 See also **Blocked or runny nose**, p.77; **Acute bronchitis**, p.104; **Heartburn**, p.107.

 ## See your doctor first

Arrange to see your doctor promptly if:

- You have breathing problems or chest pain
- You cough up blood or discolored mucus
- You are feverish and sweating
- You are losing weight
- You are taking prescribed medicine that may be causing the cough, such as certain drugs to control blood pressure

What you can do yourself

There are several things that you can do to help control a cough and to support any treatment recommended by your doctor.

- Drink at least 8 glasses of fluids a day. Include warm drinks such as soup and herbal tea, which help thin mucus and make it easier to cough up.

- To soothe your throat, try a warm honey and lemon drink (*see* NATURAL REMEDIES, p.30).

 - Normally, you shouldn't suppress a cough, since it clears the airway. However, if you have a dry, tickly cough that makes it difficult for you to sleep, try a cough suppressant (*see* DRUG REMEDIES, right).

- Warm, moist air can loosen mucus and soothe a cough. Use a humidifier, or place a bowl of water or a wet towel by a radiator. Steam inhalation may help (*see* PRACTICAL TECHNIQUE, p.79).

- Raising the head of the bed or sleeping on extra pillows may help ease a cough at night.

- Avoid smoky or dusty environments and being near people who are smoking. If you smoke, stop.

 ### DRUG REMEDIES

Cough suppressants (*see* p.180) containing dextromethorphan will help control a dry cough that keeps you awake at night or makes it difficult for you to work. Don't take cough suppressants with alcohol.

If you have a productive cough (one that brings up mucus), it is best not to take any cough mixture because coughing helps clear the mucus and irritants from the airways. (Expectorant medicines for loosening mucus are usually of little value.)

Using suppressants
Limit your use of cough suppressants during the day, because they may cause drowsiness.

 ## Seek further medical advice

Arrange to see your doctor if:

- The cough is getting worse, or it has not begun to get better after a week
- You are becoming exhausted by coughing
- The mucus becomes green, yellow, or blood-stained

Wheezing

Wheezing is a high-pitched whistling as you breathe out. Your chest may feel tight and you may find it hard to breathe. The most common cause is asthma; attacks are often an allergic reaction to inhaled substances such as dust, or are due to stress, cold air, or exercise. Other causes of wheezing include chest infection; tobacco smoke; a severe allergic reaction; or a heart or lung problem.

 See also **Hay fever**, p.80; **Anaphylactic shock**, p.159.

See your doctor first

Arrange to see your doctor promptly if you are wheezing. Check if you are taking drugs that may cause wheezing, such as anti-inflammatory analgesics or blood pressure medications.

What you can do yourself

These measures will help relieve or prevent asthma attacks, or wheezing due to other causes, and support any treatment from your doctor.

● When an asthma attack begins, try to keep calm and breathe slowly. Sit in a comfortable position; you may find it helpful to lean forward and rest your arms on a table or the back of a chair.

● If you use an asthma inhaler, keep it with you at all times and use it as directed. Keep extra inhalers at home and at work or school.

● If stress makes wheezing worse, try practicing deep breathing and muscle relaxation exercises (*see* PRACTICAL TECHNIQUES, pp.20–21). You can also use them to calm yourself during an asthma attack.

● Regular exercise, such as walking and swimming in a heated pool, can improve symptoms and keep you fit, as long as they don't make wheezing worse.

● Keep out of cold air; if you have to go out, wrap a scarf loosely around your face to warm the air as you breathe. When the air pollution level is high, stay indoors and keep doors and windows closed.

● Avoid smoky or dusty environments and allergens that might provoke an asthma attack (*see* PREVENTION, right). If you smoke, stop.

PREVENTION

Reducing allergens in the home
Many people with asthma are allergic to the droppings of dust mites. Other triggers include mold, fur and dander (flakes of skin) from pets, and household chemicals. Take these steps to reduce triggers.

● Dust surfaces with a damp cloth and try to reduce clutter in your home. Don't have too many soft toys for a child with asthma. Every 2 weeks, put them in a bag in the freezer for 6 hours, or wash with hot water.
● Use pillows and comforters with synthetic fillings, and covers that protect users from dust mites. Buy a mattress cover that fits over the whole mattress, not just the top. Wash bedding weekly at 140°F (60°C). Clean curtains regularly or replace them with blinds.
● Replace carpets with wooden or vinyl flooring, if possible, or choose short-pile synthetic carpets.
● Vacuum regularly; use a high-powered cleaner with a filter. Ask someone else to empty the machine.
● Keep your home well ventilated. Keep kitchen and bathroom doors closed to prevent dampness from spreading. Treat any mold on tiles, shower curtains, and bathroom windows with a weak bleach solution. Avoid using chemicals with strong fumes.
● If you're allergic to a pet, you may have to give it up. If you can't, keep the pet out of your bedroom completely and out of main living areas as much as possible. Have your pet groomed or bathed regularly.

Seek further medical advice

Arrange to see your doctor if:

● You cannot control asthma or other wheezing attacks using these measures

Acute bronchitis

Acute bronchitis is an infection of the airways in the lungs. It causes an irritating, persistent cough that sometimes produces thick or colored mucus (phlegm). You may also have wheezing, a fever, headache, and aches and pains. The illness is usually caused by a virus and often follows a cold. If you are otherwise healthy, it is normally not serious; you should be feeling a lot better within a few days, although the cough may linger for 3–4 weeks. You may be prone to bronchitis if you smoke or if you are exposed to pollution. People who have lung disease may have several attacks each winter.

 See also **Coughing**, p.102; **Wheezing**, p.103.

See your doctor first

Make an appointment to see your doctor if:

- You have a persistent cough and are elderly
- You have a lung condition such as asthma, or a heart problem such as heart failure
- You have difficulty breathing and chest tightness, or you are coughing up thick green, yellow, or bloodstained mucus

What you can do yourself

The following steps will help to relieve symptoms while the infection is clearing up.

- Get plenty of rest for the first few days of an attack, although you don't need to stay in bed.

- Drink at least 8 glasses of fluids a day. Warm fluids, such as soup, may be comforting.

- To soothe an irritated throat, try a warm honey and lemon drink (*see* NATURAL REMEDIES, p.30).

- Take an analgesic to reduce a temperature (*see* DRUG REMEDIES, right).

- Don't try to suppress a cough that produces mucus, since this is the body's way of clearing the airways. If you have a dry cough, however, try a cough suppressant (*see* DRUG REMEDIES, right).

- Warm, moist air loosens mucus. Use a humidifier, place a bowl of water beside a radiator to moisten the air, or sit in the bathroom while you run a bath and inhale the steam. A steam inhalation may also be helpful (*see* PRACTICAL TECHNIQUE, p.79).

- If you smoke, stop. Avoid smoky atmospheres.

DRUG REMEDIES

Analgesics such as acetaminophen (*see* p.177) or ibuprofen (*see* p.185) will reduce your temperature and help you feel more comfortable.

Cough suppressants (*see* p.180) containing dextromethorphan can help relieve a dry cough that is keeping you awake at night. Some also contain sedating antihistamines (*see* p.178) to help you sleep. Don't take suppressants with alcohol.

Sedative medicine
Cough suppressants are usually available as liquids. Some brands are useful at bedtime, because they help you sleep.

Seek further medical advice

Arrange to see your doctor if:

- You are not feeling better after 3–4 days, or the cough has not subsided within 3–4 weeks
- Breathing becomes more difficult, or you develop chest pains
- You have recurrent episodes of bronchitis

Palpitations

If you have palpitations you are suddenly aware of your heartbeat, which may feel normal, fast, or irregular. This is a common problem. Causes include exercise, excitement, stress, anxiety, and stimulants such as caffeine and nicotine. Palpitations usually occur with no other symptoms and last for a few seconds or minutes. They are normally harmless, but may be a cause for concern if they occur without obvious cause or with other symptoms, or are prolonged.

> **WARNING**
>
> Seek immediate medical help if:
> • You have palpitations and are sweaty, short of breath, have chest pain, or feel dizzy or faint
> • You suffer from an existing heart condition

 See also Panic attacks, p.24.

 ## See your doctor first

Arrange to see your doctor urgently if you have a prolonged episode of palpitations and/or frequent missed heartbeats.

What you can do yourself

If you experience occasional palpitations, try the following to help identify and deal with the cause.

● Keep a diary, noting when you have palpitations and any food or drink, exercise, stress, or other possible triggers that you have at the same time.

● If you are feeling stressed, try practicing some deep breathing and muscle relaxation exercises (*see* PRACTICAL TECHNIQUES, pp.20–21).

● Try to get plenty of sleep. Exhaustion from lack of sleep can cause or aggravate palpitations.

 ● Reduce your intake of drinks containing caffeine (*see* PRACTICAL TIPS, right). Avoid using over-the-counter stimulant pills containing caffeine.

● Before using cough or cold remedies, check the labels carefully. Some contain decongestant drugs that can cause palpitations.

● Reduce your intake of alcohol; excessive drinking is a common cause of palpitations.

● Try to give up smoking, since nicotine can speed up your heartbeat and lead to palpitations.

● Don't take illegal stimulants such as solvents, amphetamines, or cocaine, because all of these substances can cause palpitations.

PRACTICAL TIPS

Drinking less caffeine Drinks containing caffeine include coffee, tea, and cola. Reduce your intake to 2 cups a day or less, but cut down gradually; if you do it too rapidly, you may get headaches.

● Have drinks that are lower in caffeine. For example, have decaffeinated coffee, or instant coffee (which has half as much caffeine as freshly brewed coffee).
● Make coffee using half regular and half decaffeinated coffee.
● If you drink tea, brew it for less time than normal.
● Drink caffeine-free drinks such as water, fruit juice, and herbal tea.
● Check soft drink labels. Some colas, citrus-flavored drinks, and energy drinks have high caffeine levels.

 ## Seek further medical advice

Arrange to see your doctor if:

● You have recurrent episodes of palpitations despite trying to cut out possible triggers
● You develop other symptoms, such as weight loss or fatigue

Indigestion

Indigestion is stomach discomfort that usually occurs after meals, often with nausea, belching, and bloating. It is often caused by overindulgence in food or drink; stress, fatigue, or being overweight can aggravate symptoms. Sometimes, indigestion is due to a serious disorder such as a stomach ulcer or gallstones, or is a side effect of medicines such as iron supplements or certain antibiotics.

 See also **Heartburn**, opposite; **Bloating and flatulence**, p.108.

> **WARNING**
>
> Seek immediate medical help if:
> - You also have chest pain, sweating, and shortness of breath
> - You are vomiting blood or passing black stools

 ## See your doctor first

Make an appointment to see your doctor if:

- You have severe pain
- Indigestion does not seem related to eating
- You are losing weight without trying
- You are over 45 and have only recently developed indigestion

What you can do yourself

Most bouts of mild indigestion can be dealt with simply by lifestyle adjustments and home remedies.

- Try not to have foods or drinks that trigger symptoms. Familiar culprits include fatty, fried, or spicy foods, soft drinks, coffee, tea, and alcohol.

- Don't exercise for at least an hour after eating.

- If stress contributes to indigestion, try some methods that help reduce it (*see* pp.20–21).

- Stop smoking; it may aggravate symptoms.

 - Take an antacid or an H2-blocker to relieve symptoms (*see* DRUG REMEDIES, right).

- Eat at regular times. You're less likely to get indigestion if you eat smaller meals more often. Eat slowly, chewing your food thoroughly.

- Avoid taking aspirin or ibuprofen for pain, as they can irritate the stomach. Acetaminophen (*see* p.177) may be a more suitable alternative.

 - Try a herbal tea to soothe your stomach (*see* NATURAL REMEDIES, right).

- If you are overweight, try to lose weight gradually.

 ### DRUG REMEDIES

Antacids (*see* p.177) can relieve indigestion by neutralizing acid in the stomach. Some antacid combinations contain simethicone to absorb excess stomach gas. If you are taking other medication, avoid taking antacids at the same time as antacids may reduce its absorption.

H2-blockers (*see* p.183) reduce acid produced by the stomach. Try a short course (not more than 2 weeks) of cimetidine or ranitidine if antacids are not effective.

Antacids
Liquids are more effective; pills may be more convenient.

 ### NATURAL REMEDIES

Herbal tea (*see* p.184) made with peppermint, chamomile, or fennel may help to relieve the symptoms of indigestion.

Seek further medical advice

Arrange to see your doctor if:

- Your symptoms become worse
- Symptoms are not improving after a week or two
- You have recurrent indigestion

Heartburn

Heartburn is a burning feeling that starts in your lower chest and stomach and may rise to your throat. You may have a bitter taste in your mouth, and feel sick and bloated. Some people have a dry cough, especially at night. Heartburn often occurs after a heavy meal, and is more likely if you lie down or bend over. It is due to acid reflux, in which stomach acid leaks into the esophagus.

 See also **Indigestion**, opposite page.

WARNING

Seek immediate medical help if:
- You have prolonged chest pain, sweating, and shortness of breath
- You are vomiting blood or passing black stools
- You have difficulty swallowing

What you can do yourself

You should be able to prevent or relieve episodes of heartburn with the following measures.

- Avoid foods likely to trigger heartburn, such as citrus fruits, chocolate, spicy and fatty foods, coffee, and tomatoes. Avoid alcoholic or very hot drinks.

- Try not to bend or stoop over. Don't sit hunched up at your desk; this will encourage heartburn.

- Don't wear tight-fitting clothes or belts.

- Stop smoking; it may aggravate heartburn.

 - Take an antacid or H2-blocker to relieve the symptoms (*see* DRUG REMEDIES, right).

- Eat small, regular meals rather than occasional big meals. Don't eat within 2 or 3 hours of bedtime.

- Avoid analgesics or cold remedies that contain aspirin or ibuprofen; they may aggravate heartburn.

 - Try a soothing herbal tea to help relieve heartburn (*see* NATURAL REMEDIES, opposite page).

 - Sleep with your head raised to help prevent acid reflux (*see* PRACTICAL TIP, right).

- If you are overweight, try to lose weight gradually to ease pressure on your stomach.

Seek medical advice

Arrange to see your doctor if:

- Your symptoms become worse, or do not improve after a week or two
- You are getting recurrent bouts of heartburn

DRUG REMEDIES

Antacids (*see* p.177) neutralize stomach acid, providing quick relief for occasional, mild episodes of heartburn. If you are taking other medication, avoid taking antacids at the same time as antacids may reduce its absorption.

H2-blockers (*see* p.183) work by reducing acid in the stomach. If antacids are not effective, try a short course (not more than 2 weeks) of a medicine containing cimetidine or ranitidine.

PRACTICAL TIP

Sleep with your head raised

To help prevent stomach acid leaking back into your esophagus at night, keep your head higher than your body. Prop up the head of your bed 4–6 in (10–15 cm). If you nap during the day, sleep upright in a chair.

Raising the bed head
Sturdy, solid objects, such as bricks or pieces of wood, placed under the head of the bed help to keep your head raised.

Bloating and flatulence

A bloated abdomen and flatulence (gas) are common complaints, caused by a buildup of excess gas in your digestive system. You may also experience sharp pains and rumbling noises in your abdomen. Most cases of bloating and flatulence are due to food, particularly foods such as beans and cabbage, which produce gas as they are digested. Eating too fast can also cause excessive gas. Certain people find that milk, food additives, or wheat flour can produce symptoms. Sometimes, bloating and flatulence are due to a bowel disorder such as irritable bowel syndrome.

 See also Irritable bowel syndrome, p.111; Food intolerance, p.113.

See your doctor first

Make an appointment to see your doctor if you also have other bowel symptoms, such as constipation, diarrhea, blood in your stools, nausea, vomiting, or continual or recurrent abdominal pains.

What you can do yourself

Try these measures to prevent a buildup of gas or to treat bloating and flatulence.

● Try to identify and cut down on any foods that cause problems. The worst offenders include cabbage, cauliflower, brussels sprouts, onions, garlic, prunes, raisins, beans, and spicy foods.

● You may develop gas or bloating if you add high-fiber foods to your diet too quickly. Reduce your intake, then increase it gradually over 2–3 weeks.

● Eat and drink slowly, and chew food thoroughly. You may find it helps to eat several small meals a day instead of one or two large ones.

● Cut down on beer and carbonated drinks; chewing gum; smoking; and the artificial sweeteners sorbitol and mannitol (found in some sugar-free sweet foods). All of these things may contribute to flatulence.

 ● Preparations containing simethicone can be used to treat flatulence (*see* DRUG REMEDIES, right).

 ● Try drinking herbal tea to relieve symptoms (*see* NATURAL REMEDIES, right).

DRUG REMEDIES

Simethicone (*see* FLATULENCE RELIEF, p.183) helps to disperse excess gas. It is usually combined with an antacid, or sometimes with activated charcoal, as an indigestion remedy. If you are taking other medication, avoid taking antacids at the same time as antacids may reduce its absorption.

NATURAL REMEDIES

Herbal teas (*see* p.184) made with chamomile, peppermint, or fennel may help to calm a bloated stomach and relieve excess gas.

Soothing tea
Sip soothing herbal tea to help relieve digestive problems.

 ## Seek further medical advice

Arrange to see your doctor if bloating and flatulence persist after 2 weeks or new symptoms develop.

Nausea and vomiting

There are many reasons for nausea. The mere sight or smell of something unpleasant, or a food you dislike, may trigger sweating and queasiness. Anxiety and motion sickness are also common causes. Nausea doesn't always lead to vomiting; if it does, it is often due to gastroenteritis (an infection), food poisoning, or excess alcohol. Morning sickness is common in early pregnancy, and migraine sufferers may vomit during attacks. Nausea and vomiting are usually short-lived, but repeated vomiting may dehydrate you.

WARNING

Seek immediate medical help if nausea and vomiting follow a head injury or are accompanied by:
- Blood in the vomit
- Severe headache or stiff neck
- Severe abdominal pain

See your doctor first

Arrange to see your doctor if you can't establish the cause of your nausea or vomiting.

What you can do yourself

Try these measures to help you recover quickly from nausea and/or vomiting and prevent dehydration.

- If you feel nauseated, open a window or step outside for a few minutes to get some fresh air.

- Drink at least 8 glasses of clear fluids, such as water or apple juice, each day. Sip slowly. Avoid drinks that can irritate the stomach, such as alcohol, coffee, and cola, and avoid drinking during a meal. Passing small volumes of dark urine shows you are becoming dehydrated and need to drink more.

- If you can, eat small, frequent meals. Eat slowly. Start with bland foods such as boiled rice, pasta, chicken soup, or dry toast. Avoid spicy and oily foods and very hot or very cold foods and drinks.

- Try to rest after meals; sit in a chair or propped up in bed (lying flat may make you feel worse). Don't move around too much, as this can lead to vomiting.

- Avoid strong odors such as perfumes, since they can provoke vomiting.

- Taking ginger (*see* NATURAL REMEDIES, right) may relieve nausea, especially motion sickness.

- If you have morning sickness, keep plain crackers by your bed and eat one just before you get up.

- Take an oral rehydration preparation if you have been vomiting (*see* DRUG REMEDIES, right).

DRUG REMEDIES

Oral rehydration solutions (*see* p.188) replace salts, sugar, and minerals that have been lost from your body through vomiting. They are available as ready-to-use bottled solutions in a variety of flavors. Sip them instead of, or in addition to, regular drinks.

NATURAL REMEDIES

Ginger (*see* p.183) can be soothing during a bout of nausea and is a useful treatment for motion sickness (*see* p.110). You can take ginger root capsules; alternatively, eat some pieces of crystallized or raw ginger, add powdered ginger to a glass of fruit juice, or make ginger tea.

Seek further medical advice

Arrange to see your doctor if:

- Your nausea or vomiting doesn't start to subside within 24 hours
- You develop any other symptoms
- You are taking regular medication, such as birth control pills, because vomiting may reduce its effectiveness

Motion sickness

If you suffer from motion sickness, or travel sickness, you will have feelings of nausea and dizziness, and possibly a headache, whenever you travel by car, ship, train, or plane. If the motion continues, you begin to feel worse and may break out in a sweat, breathe rapidly and shallowly, turn pale, and vomit. Motion sickness occurs when your brain receives conflicting messages from the balance organs inside the ears and from the eyes. Some people are more susceptible to motion sickness than others, and anxiety can contribute to the problem. Children are generally more prone to the condition than adults.

What you can do yourself

There are several measures that help to prevent or minimize motion sickness. Plan how to put them into effect before you start your trip.

- Before you travel, eat a little bland food. Avoid having alcohol and carbonated drinks before and during your trip.

- Try taking motion sickness pills before traveling (*see* DRUG REMEDIES, right).

- On board a vehicle, try to choose a position with the least motion. In a plane, sit halfway down, by a window overlooking the wings. In a ship, sit in the middle, or stay on deck if you can. If you are below deck or in an enclosed cabin, try to sleep as much as you can. In a train, sit by a window, facing the direction of travel. In a car, sit in a front seat.

- Make sure that you have access to fresh air. Avoid strong odors and cigarette smoke.

- In a car or train, focus on the horizon or something in the distance in the direction of travel. Avoid reading, writing, or looking down.

- Eating some ginger may help to relieve nausea (*see* NATURAL REMEDIES, right).

- You may find that traveling at night reduces sickness, particularly if you manage to sleep.

- If anxiety plays a part, try exercises to control your breathing (*see* PRACTICAL TECHNIQUE, p.20).

- Try acupressure bands. They are thought to relieve nausea by stimulating a point on the wrist.

- If your child has motion sickness, use a booster seat so that he or she can look out the window. Distract your child with music, a story tape or CD, or games that involve looking for things ahead.

DRUG REMEDIES

Motion sickness pills (*see* p.187) contain antihistamines, such as meclizine or dimenhydrinate, which help control symptoms. Take them before you start a trip. They may make you drowsy, so don't drive after taking them. They may also increase the effects of alcohol, so avoid alcoholic drinks once you have taken them.

NATURAL REMEDIES

Ginger (*see* p.183) has been shown to reduce symptoms of motion sickness. Take ginger root capsules an hour or two before you start a trip. Alternatively, try nibbling a slice of fresh ginger or crystallized ginger, or taking ½–1 teaspoon of powdered ginger in fruit juice. A child may prefer a ginger cookie or candy.

Ginger root and powder
Eat fresh ginger or stir powdered ginger into fruit juice.

 ### Seek medical advice

Arrange to see your doctor if:

- You still have motion sickness symptoms a day or two after travel
- You have symptoms such as nausea and dizziness when you are not traveling

Irritable bowel syndrome

Symptoms of irritable bowel syndrome (IBS) vary. The most common are bloating, abdominal pain, and cramps, which ease after you pass gas or a bowel motion. You may have loose stools or constipation, or alternate between the two; notice mucus in your stools; and have the feeling that your bowel has not emptied after a bowel movement. You may feel full more quickly than normal during meals. Other symptoms include nausea, back pain, frequent urination, and headaches. Although symptoms are intermittent, IBS may last for years. The cause is not known, but sensitivity to certain foods, bowel infection, and stress can trigger attacks.

 See also Stress, pp.20–21; Bloating and flatulence, p.108; Constipation, p.115; Diarrhea, p.116.

See your doctor first

Make an appointment to see your doctor if you think you have IBS. Other causes need to be ruled out, because symptoms of IBS are similar to those of more serious bowel conditions.

What you can do yourself

Try the following changes to your diet and lifestyle to see what works best for you.

- Keep a food diary for 2 or 3 weeks to identify any triggers. Common triggers for IBS include dairy products, wheat, citrus fruits, alcohol, and coffee.

- Eat and drink slowly, and chew food thoroughly. It may help to eat several small meals a day.

 - If constipation is a problem, gradually add more fiber to your diet, such as cereals, whole-grain bread, brown rice, beans, fruit, and vegetables. Avoid unprocessed bran since it can make symptoms worse. Try fiber supplements (*see* DRUG REMEDIES, right).

- If you have diarrhea, cut down on tea, coffee, cola, alcohol, and oily foods, and stop smoking. Drink 6–8 glasses of water a day; no carbonated drinks.

 - If you are troubled by abdominal pain or bloating, try peppermint oil (*see* NATURAL REMEDIES, right).

- Walk, cycle, or swim for 20–30 minutes a day to help reduce stress and regulate the bowels.

- If stress triggers IBS, practice exercises to help you relax (*see* PRACTICAL TECHNIQUES, pp.20–21).

- If lifestyle changes don't help diarrhea, try antidiarrheal drugs (*see* DRUG REMEDIES, right).

NATURAL REMEDIES

Peppermint oil (*see* p.188) works by relaxing the bowel muscle, helping to relieve abdominal pain and bloating.

DRUG REMEDIES

Fiber supplements (*see* LAXATIVES, p.185) contain fiber derived from plants. They can help if you are prone to constipation and are finding it difficult to include extra fiber in your diet. Consult your doctor before taking fiber supplements.

Antidiarrheal drugs (*see* p.178) containing loperamide can be used to help control diarrhea for a limited time, such as during a long car trip. Take the lowest

Taking fiber supplements
Mix the fiber supplement in half a glass of water and drink it immediately.

 ## Seek further medical advice

Arrange to see your doctor if:

- Your symptoms worsen or do not subside after 2 weeks of following the self-help measures given on this page
- You develop new symptoms

Hernia

A hernia is a lump in the groin or, less commonly, at the navel, that tends to disappear when you lie flat. In men, a hernia may appear in the scrotum. You may have no other symptoms, or may feel pain or a dragging sensation. Hernias occur when part of the intestine pushes through a weak spot in your abdominal muscles. They are often due to increased pressure in the abdomen as a result of activities such as heavy lifting, coughing, sneezing, or straining on the toilet. Being overweight makes you more susceptible.

WARNING

Seek urgent medical help if:

● You have a hernia that you can't gently push back in and/or you have heat and tenderness over the lump; nausea and vomiting; severe abdominal pain; and constipation

 ## See your doctor first

Arrange to see your doctor to confirm that you have a hernia and to discuss treatment.

What you can do yourself

A hernia usually requires surgery, but there are several things you can do that will support treatment from your doctor.

 ● If your work involves heavy lifting, try to arrange lighter duties. Once you are better, take care with lifting heavy objects (*see* PREVENTION, right).

● Eat a high-fiber diet with plenty of fruit, vegetables, and whole-grain bread, and drink 6–8 glasses of water a day; this will help keep your bowel movements regular. Avoid straining when you are on the toilet.

● Stop smoking, because a smoker's cough puts pressure on a hernia.

● Lose any excess weight, because the weight puts a strain on your abdominal wall.

● Wearing a groin support is of only limited value unless the device has been fitted properly on the advice of a doctor.

Seek further medical help

Arrange to see your doctor again if:

● The hernia gets larger and more painful while you're waiting for treatment

PREVENTION

Lifting heavy objects The following technique may help prevent another hernia, particularly if your job involves heavy manual work. If an object feels too heavy, don't try to lift or move it without a lifting aid, wheel base, or cart.

1 *When you lift a heavy object, bend your knees (not your back) and use your leg muscles to provide the lifting power. Squat close to the object and grasp it at the base.*

Keep your back straight and avoid twisting

2 *Straighten your knees and push yourself up with your leg muscles in one smooth movement.*

3 *When you are carrying an object, keep the weight close to your body, your back straight, and your head up. When you put the object down, bend at the knees.*

Keep the weight balanced over your thighs and feet

Food intolerance

If you have symptoms such as bloating, abdominal pain, diarrhea, or nausea each time you eat a certain food, you may be "intolerant," or unable to digest it properly. The most likely triggers are dairy products and cereals (such as wheat). Food intolerance is distinct from food allergy, which is less common but in some people can cause a life-threatening reaction called anaphylactic shock.

 See also **Bloating and flatulence**, p.108; **Diarrhea**, p.116; **Anaphylactic shock**, p.159.

> ## WARNING
> Seek immediate medical help if:
> ● You develop breathing difficulties, swelling of your lips and tongue, and a rash within a few minutes of eating a suspect food

See your doctor first

Make an appointment to see your doctor if:

● You think you may be intolerant to wheat, rye, barley, and possibly oats (gluten intolerance, also called celiac disease) or of milk and other dairy products (lactose intolerance)
● You have symptoms such as weight loss

What you can do yourself

The following advice will help you identify and treat mild food intolerance; use it alongside any advice from your doctor.

 ● Try to identify the food causing your symptoms (*see* PRACTICAL TECHNIQUE, right).

● If your doctor has diagnosed lactose intolerance, avoid dairy products. Try soy milk or other milk substitutes, which are now available in many supermarkets. Check for hidden lactose in foods such as cookies. You may also wish to try a lactase supplement (*see* DRUG REMEDIES, right).

● If you are diagnosed as having gluten intolerance (celiac disease), cut cereals, bread, pasta, cakes, and cookies out of your diet. Check for hidden gluten in processed foods such as ice cream and canned soup; candies; and medicines. Many supermarkets and health food shops sell gluten-free pastas, breads, and other foods.

● Check labels on food packaging for the food or additive to which you're intolerant. This may not always be obvious: for example, "casein" is milk protein, and "albumin" is egg white.

PRACTICAL TECHNIQUE

Elimination diet If you think you may have a food intolerance, take these steps to find the trigger.

● Keep a diary for 2–3 weeks, noting what you eat and drink and how much, and when symptoms occur. (Symptoms can develop from a few hours to a few days after exposure to a trigger substance.)
● Exclude a suspect substance from your diet for a week or two. If symptoms return when you reintroduce the item, you may be intolerant of it.
● If you find a specific trigger, avoid it. However, if you think you are affected by a whole group of foods, such as dairy or wheat products, see your doctor first.

DRUG REMEDIES

Lactase supplements (*see* p.185), usually available in tablet form, help break down lactose in dairy foods. They are useful if you are lactose intolerant and find it difficult to limit your milk intake, or if you develop symptoms after having even small amounts of dairy products. Take the supplement just before you consume dairy products.

Seek further medical advice

Arrange to see your doctor if:

● Your symptoms don't improve after using the measures described above
● You develop any new symptoms, such as weight loss

Food poisoning

Most attacks of food poisoning are due to poor hygiene, cooking, or food storage, which allows bacteria or viruses in contaminated food to multiply. The most commonly affected foods are seafood, dairy products, and undercooked eggs and poultry. Symptoms of food poisoning include nausea, vomiting, diarrhea, and cramps in the abdomen, and, sometimes, fever, headache, and dizziness.

 See also **Nausea and vomiting,** p.109; **Diarrhea,** p.116.

WARNING

Seek immediate medical help if:
● You suffer from blurred vision and muscle weakness after eating contaminated food

 ## See your doctor first

Make an appointment to see your doctor if:

● You have severe abdominal pain or vomiting
● There is blood or mucus in your stools

What you can do yourself

You can treat a mild case of food poisoning at home using the following measures. You should feel better within a day or two.

● Get plenty of rest and make yourself as comfortable as possible.

 ● Drink at least 8 glasses of clear fluids a day. Take small sips so that you don't vomit. If necessary, drink an oral rehydration solution (*see* DRUG REMEDIES, right).

● As soon as you can eat, have bland foods such as boiled rice, pasta, and mashed potatoes. Start with small amounts, returning to your normal diet once you can eat these foods without problems. You should avoid tea, coffee, dairy products, alcohol, and fatty or spicy foods until a few days after the diarrhea has stopped.

● Be careful about hygiene to avoid passing on the infection to other people. Wash your hands thoroughly after going to the bathroom, and have your own towel. Don't make food for others, or share utensils, cups, or plates. Keep away from those who are vulnerable to infections, such as young children, elderly people, and pregnant women.

 ● Take an antidiarrheal medicine if you need to stop diarrhea quickly (*see* DRUG REMEDIES, right).

 ## DRUG REMEDIES

Oral rehydration solutions (*see* p.188) replace salts, sugar, and minerals that have been lost from your body. They are available as ready-to-use solutions in a variety of flavors. Have them instead of, or in addition to, regular drinks.

Antidiarrheal drugs (*see* p.178) should be used only as a last resort because diarrhea is the body's way of getting rid of infection. You can take loperamide for quick relief if diarrhea is likely to cause embarrassment, for example, at work.

 ## PREVENTION

Food hygiene Follow these steps to prevent germs from multiplying and avoid food poisoning.

● Before preparing food, wash your hands with warm water and soap, and dry them on a clean hand towel.
● Keep raw and prepared foods separate. Store raw meat in the bottom of the refrigerator to prevent drips.
● Use different chopping boards and work surfaces for raw meat, cooked meat, and vegetables. Clean boards and surfaces thoroughly after use.
● Cook food thoroughly, especially meat, fish, or eggs.
● When reheating food, ensure that it is very hot all the way through. Don't reheat it more than once.

 ## Seek further medical advice

Arrange to see your doctor if your symptoms are getting worse or have not cleared up within 28–48 hours.

Constipation

The normal frequency of bowel movements can vary from 3 times a day to 3 times a week, and most people have a regular habit. However, if you pass hard stools less than 3 times a week, you are probably constipated. Other symptoms include bloating, nausea, and cramping in your lower abdomen. Eating a diet that is low in fiber, not drinking enough fluids, having a sedentary lifestyle, and/or repeatedly ignoring the urge to go to the bathroom can contribute to constipation. Some medicines, such as certain analgesics and iron supplements, may cause or aggravate the problem. Occasionally, constipation is caused by an underlying illness.

See your doctor first

Arrange to see your doctor if you have unexplained changes in your bowel habit, or:

- You are passing blood, mucus, or pus
- You have severe pain in your abdomen
- You are losing weight

What you can do yourself

There are various ways to treat a mild bout of constipation and prevent it from recurring.

- Some foods, such as prunes and figs, have natural laxative properties, so include these with your meals. Don't skip breakfast. Having a hot drink with breakfast helps to stimulate the bowels.

- Drink at least 8 glasses of water and/or fruit juice a day. Cut down on tea, coffee, and cola, which can make you dehydrated.

- Try to get 20–30 minutes of exercise, such as walking, cycling, or swimming, every day, since activity helps stimulate the bowels.

- If other measures have not helped, try taking a fiber supplement (*see* NATURAL REMEDIES, right).

- Use a stimulant laxative if constipation is severe or persistent (*see* DRUG REMEDIES, right).

Seek further medical advice

Arrange to see your doctor if:

- Constipation has not cleared up after 7 days
- You have not had a normal bowel movement but have had leakage of feces or diarrhea
- You get recurrent bouts of constipation

NATURAL REMEDIES

Fiber supplements (*see* LAXATIVES, p.185) make stools softer, bulkier, and easier to pass. The most common type is bran, which can be mixed with cereal, soup, or fruit juice. Start with a small amount and increase gradually. If bran is unpalatable, try a product containing methylcellulose.

DRUG REMEDIES

Stimulant laxatives (*see* LAXATIVES, p.185), such as senna, can be used for temporary relief, but long-term or excessive use of stimulant laxatives may make you more constipated because your bowels no longer move efficiently without them.

PREVENTION

Avoiding constipation The following measures will ensure that constipation doesn't recur.

- Go to the bathroom when you have the urge; don't wait. Allow adequate time for bowel movements.
- Increase your fiber intake by gradually adding foods such as muesli, whole-grain bread, vegetables, and nuts to your diet. Drink plenty of fluids with the fiber.

Healthy breakfast
Add fresh fruit to muesli for a high-fiber breakfast.

Diarrhea

During an attack of diarrhea, you pass loose or watery feces frequently. You may also lose your appetite and have vomiting, abdominal cramps, bloating, and a headache. If the problem continues, you can become dehydrated due to the loss of large amounts of fluids and salts from your body. Diarrhea is normally caused by bacteria or viruses found in infected food or transmitted from one person to another. In addition, some drugs, such as antibiotics, can cause short-term diarrhea. An episode of diarrhea normally clears up within a few days, but ongoing or recurrent diarrhea can indicate an underlying bowel condition.

 See also Food intolerance, p.113; Food poisoning, p.114.

 See your doctor first

Make an appointment to see your doctor if:

- You have severe pain in your abdomen and/or you are vomiting
- You notice blood or mucus in your feces

What you can do yourself

A mild episode of diarrhea will clear up on its own in a few days. The following steps will ease symptoms and help prevent dehydration.

- Drink at least 8 glasses a day of clear liquids such as water, weak tea, thin soups, and fruit juice. If you are vomiting, have a drink beside you all the time and take frequent small sips. Passing small volumes of dark urine indicates that you are becoming dehydrated and need to drink more.

 • Try taking an oral rehydration solution (*see* DRUG REMEDIES, right).

• Gradually start eating again as soon as you feel able. Start with bland foods such as boiled rice, pasta, mashed potatoes, and dry toast. Avoid tea, coffee, and cola, dairy products, alcohol, and fatty and spicy foods while you have diarrhea and for a few days after it has cleared up.

 • It is best to let diarrhea run its course because it is the body's way of eliminating infection. You can, however, use antidiarrheal drugs as a short-term solution when you are out, at work, or going on a long trip (*see* DRUG REMEDIES, right).

 • Take an analgesic if you have fever or headaches with the diarrhea (*see* DRUG REMEDIES, right).

DRUG REMEDIES

Oral rehydration solutions (*see* p.188) replace water, sugars, and salts lost from the body during an attack of diarrhea. They are available as ready-to-use bottled solutions. Drink them instead of, or in addition to, regular drinks.

Antidiarrheal drugs (*see* p.178) contain loperamide and work by slowing down bowel activity. Usually, 2 capsules are taken immediately, followed by 1 capsule after each loose stool. Don't take more than 8 capsules in 24 hours.

Analgesics Acetaminophen (*see* p.177) will help reduce fever and discomfort and is less likely to irritate your bowels than other analgesics.

Oral rehydration *Bottled rehydration solutions come in a range of flavors.*

 Seek further medical advice

Arrange to see your doctor if:

- The diarrhea gets worse
- There is no improvement in 24–48 hours

Hemorrhoids

Hemorrhoids are swollen veins that develop in or around the anus. They mainly affect people who are constipated, who frequently strain when having a bowel movement, or have repeated episodes of diarrhea. The most common symptom is bright red blood on toilet paper or in the toilet bowl. Opening your bowels may be painful and it may feel as if they have not emptied completely. Sitting down may be uncomfortable. The skin around your anus may be itchy and irritated. Hemorrhoids can also protrude outside the anus and form a painful swelling. The condition is more common in pregnant women and overweight people.

 See also **Constipation**, p.115; **Diarrhea**, opposite page; **Itchy anus**, p.118.

 ## See your doctor first

Make an appointment to see your doctor if:

- You have bleeding from your anus and/or a lump inside or near the anus

What you can do yourself

Hemorrhoids can be uncomfortable, but there are measures that you can take to help relieve them and support any treatment from your doctor.

- Treat constipation promptly to avoid triggering or aggravating hemorrhoids. Small hemorrhoids often subside once constipation is relieved.

- Go to the bathroom as soon as you feel the need. Don't strain or hold your breath when having a bowel movement, and don't rush. Even if it feels as if you have not emptied your bowels, resist the urge to strain at the end of a bowel movement.

- Clean your anal area after each bowel movement with a moist cloth or unscented, moist toilet tissue.

- If possible, sit in a shallow, warm bath for about 15 minutes, 3 or 4 times a day. Don't use soap to wash your anal area. Pat the area dry afterward.

 - Take an analgesic to reduce the discomfort (*see* DRUG REMEDIES, right).

- If you have a painful, protruding hemorrhoid, rest in bed for a day. Apply an ice pack (a bag of crushed ice or frozen vegetables, wrapped in a wet towel) to the anus for 15–20 minutes up to 4 times a day.

 - Try an over-the-counter hemorrhoid preparation (*see* DRUG REMEDIES, right).

 ### DRUG REMEDIES

Analgesics Taking acetaminophen (*see* p.177) or ibuprofen (*see* p.185) can help relieve the discomfort of hemorrhoids. If the pain persists for more than a few days, however, stop taking the analgesics and consult your doctor.

Hemorrhoid preparations (*see* p.184) are available as creams, ointments, pads, and suppositories. They soothe painful hemorrhoids and make it easier to have bowel movements. They may contain phenylephrine, which shrinks swollen tissue, witch hazel to relieve itching and irritation, or hydrocortisone to reduce inflammation. Don't use hemorrhoid preparations for longer than 6 days since you may develop a reaction to the ingredients.

Creams and suppositories
Use an applicator to apply the cream; insert suppositories into the anus.

 ## Seek further medical advice

Arrange to see your doctor if:

- The bleeding gets worse
- Bleeding, irritation, or pain does not subside after a few days of treatment

Itchy anus

Anal itching is uncomfortable and may be embarrassing because you will have a strong urge to scratch. The skin around your anus may be red and sore, and may bleed and become infected if you scratch a great deal. Itching is often worse after emptying your bowels, and at night. In most cases, an itchy anus is due to irritation from toiletries, or from sweat, moisture, or traces of feces left in contact with the skin. People who are overweight, sweat profusely, and/or wear tight-fitting underwear are more susceptible. Sometimes a particular food contributes to the problem. Hemorrhoids and pinworms are common causes of itching.

 See also Hemorrhoids, p.117; Pinworms, p.137.

 ## See your doctor first

Make an appointment to see your doctor if:

- You have anal bleeding or a mucus discharge
- You have pain and/or a lump near your anus

What you can do yourself

Anal itching can usually be relieved with home treatment, which may also help prevent recurrences.

- Resist the urge to scratch. Cut your fingernails short and wear cotton gloves at night.

 • Try a sedative antihistamine to reduce itching and help you sleep (*see* DRUG REMEDIES, right).

- Wash your anus morning and evening with plain water and pat the area dry. Make sure the area is completely dry – using a hair dryer may be helpful.

 • Applying a hemorrhoid cream or witch hazel pad after washing may soothe itching (*see* DRUG REMEDIES, right). Alternatively, use calendula cream (*see* NATURAL REMEDIES, right).

- Wash after each bowel movement. When this is not possible, use a moistened cloth or unscented, moist toilet tissues. Use plain toilet tissue after urinating to dry yourself thoroughly.

- Wear loose cotton underwear, and change it daily or more often if necessary. Avoid wearing tight-fitting pants or pantyhose. A strip of cotton or tissue next to your anus will absorb moisture.

- Try to identify and then cut down on food or drink that may be contributing to anal itching, such as beer, coffee, tomatoes, or spicy foods.

 ## DRUG REMEDIES

Antihistamines (*see* p.178) relieve itching. Taking a sedative antihistamine, available as pills or liquid medicine, will also help you sleep.

Hemorrhoid preparations (*see* p.184) may contain phenylephrine, which shrinks swollen tissue, witch hazel to relieve itching and irritation, or hydrocortisone to reduce inflammation. Don't use them for longer than 5–6 days.

 ## NATURAL REMEDIES

Calendula cream (*see* p.179) is a mild, soothing cream made from extracts of the calendula (pot marigold) plant. Apply it once a day after washing. Discontinue if you develop a reaction to the cream.

Using calendula
Apply calendula cream sparingly and rub it in lightly.

 ## Seek further medical advice

Arrange to see your doctor if:

- The itchiness does not subside after about a week of using the above measures
- You develop any new symptoms or other family members develop an itch

MEN'S PROBLEMS

Painful scrotum

Minor injury to the scrotum does not usually cause lasting harm, but sudden severe pain can be due to torsion (twisting) of one of the testes inside, which can cause permanent damage. A painful, tender scrotum, sometimes with swelling, may be due to an infection (epididymitis). You may also have a fever and pain when urinating. Other causes of pain include mumps and, rarely, testicular cancer.

 See also Mumps, p.26.

> ### WARNING
> Seek immediate medical help if:
> - You develop sudden or severe pain in the scrotum
> - Pain after an injury to the area persists for more than an hour

 ## See your doctor first

Arrange to see your doctor promptly if:

- You have had mild pain for more than 2 days
- You think you have epididymitis
- You find a lump in the scrotum or testes

What you can do yourself

Try the following home treatments alone or in conjunction with treatment from your doctor.

- To relieve pain and swelling, apply an ice pack (such as a bag of frozen peas or crushed ice in a plastic bag wrapped in a wet towel) to the testes. Hold for about 10 minutes. Use twice a day. You can also take an analgesic (*see* DRUG REMEDIES, right).

- Lie on your back with a rolled-up towel placed between your legs and under the scrotum to lift it and relieve discomfort. When moving around, wear an athletic support or two pairs of close-fitting underpants, especially if the testes are swollen.

- When the pain has eased, check your testes regularly for lumps (*see* PRACTICAL TECHNIQUE, right).

 ## Seek further medical advice

Arrange to see your doctor if:

- The pain is worse or no better after 2 days

DRUG REMEDIES

Analgesics can be used to reduce pain and swelling in the scrotum and also fever. Take an anti-inflammatory analgesic such as ibuprofen (*see* p.185).

PRACTICAL TECHNIQUE

Testicular self-examination All men should examine their testes regularly to detect lumps or other changes that may be an early sign of cancer.

- Examine yourself once a month after a warm bath, when the scrotum is relaxed. Check for any lumps or swellings. Both testes should be smooth except along the top and back, where you will feel a soft tube (epididymis) that carries and stores sperm.
- Compare one testis with the other if you are not sure whether one feels normal (it is unusual to develop cancer in both testes at the same time). If you notice any changes in either your testes or your scrotum, consult your doctor promptly.

Examining your testes
Carefully roll your fingers and thumb across the entire surface of each testis in turn.

Painful penis

The skin on the penis is thin and delicate and is easily injured or irritated. Minor bruising and chafing may occur after playing sports or sexual activity. Soreness at the tip may be due to poor hygiene or irritation from soaps or spermicides, or result from infections, including sexually transmitted infections (STDs). Other symptoms of an STD include a rash, discharge from the penis, and pain when urinating. Pain that occurs only when your penis is erect or during sex may be due to an overtight foreskin.

> ### WARNING
> Seek immediate medical help if:
> - You have a painful erection that lasts long after arousal has passed
> - You have difficulty rolling your foreskin forward again after it has been retracted

See your doctor first

Arrange to see your doctor, or go to a sexually transmitted disease clinic if:

- You suspect that you have a sexually transmitted disease or you are not sure what is causing the pain

What you can do yourself

There are several measures you can take that will ease pain and help prevent soreness.

- Keep your penis and foreskin clean. Take a bath or shower every day. If you have a foreskin, wash underneath it with water and unperfumed soap. Dry the end of your penis thoroughly.

- Wear loose underwear to avoid discomfort.

- If the head of your penis gets inflamed or sore during sex, apply a water-soluble lubricating jelly beforehand (*see* DRUG REMEDIES, right). Wash your genitals after intercourse. If you think the problem is due to the condoms you use, switch to a nonlatex type or one with a different spermicide.

- If you have a small injury on the tip of your penis, let it heal completely before having sex again.

- If you think you may be sensitive to soaps and laundry detergents, use only nonallergenic powder for your underclothes and avoid fabric softeners.

- If you have a sexually transmitted infection, bathing with salt water will help relieve symptoms (*see* PRACTICAL TIP, right). Tell your partner you have an STD; he or she may also need treatment.

DRUG REMEDIES

Lubricating jelly (*see* p.186) is widely available and will make sex more comfortable. Use it to help prevent soreness that may develop because of irritants or vigorous activity.

Using jelly
Apply a water-soluble lubricant to your penis just before intercourse.

PRACTICAL TIP

Salt-water baths Gently bathing your penis 2 or 3 times a day in warm, salty water will help relieve soreness, swelling, and inflammation. Add a handful of salt to a bath two-thirds full. If you are finding urination uncomfortable or painful, urinate while lying in a warm bath, and shower yourself and the bathtub afterward.

Seek further medical advice

Arrange to see your doctor or go to a urologist if:

- Pain in your penis persists, or you develop new symptoms

Urinary problems in men

Many urinary problems in men that start in later life are due to enlargement of the prostate gland, which lies beneath the bladder. This condition is usually noncancerous (in which case it is called benign prostatic hyperplasia), but sometimes it is due to cancer. The prostate may constrict the bladder outlet, causing symptoms such as an urgent or frequent need to urinate (including at night); a weak flow; dribbling afterward; and a feeling that your bladder has not emptied completely.

WARNING

Seek immediate medical help if:
- You develop pain or swelling in your abdomen and can't urinate

See your doctor first

Make an appointment to see your doctor if:

- You have problems when urinating, especially if there is blood in the urine or you feel a burning sensation
- You are taking an over-the-counter or prescribed medicine that may be making the problem worse, such as a decongestant or an antidepressant

What you can do yourself

Use these self-help measures alongside treatment from your doctor to help minimize urinary problems.

- Drink 6–8 glasses of fluid a day so your urine doesn't get too concentrated and cause irritation. Avoid drinking too much over a short time, however, since this may cause a sudden urge to urinate.

- Urinate only when your bladder feels full. Take your time so that your bladder empties completely. Sometimes sitting on the toilet is more effective.

- If you often need to get up at night, drink less in the evening and stop drinking a few hours before bedtime. Empty your bladder before going to bed.

- Reduce your intake of tea, coffee, cola, and alcohol. These drinks make your bladder fill quickly and cause a sudden or urgent need to urinate.

- Avoid carbonated drinks, citrus fruits and juices, and spicy foods, since they may irritate your bladder.

- Try saw palmetto if you have benign prostate enlargement (*see* NATURAL REMEDIES, right).

NATURAL REMEDIES

Saw palmetto (*see* p.188) tinctures and supplements are made from the berries of the saw palmetto plant. You can take them to improve urine flow and bladder emptying if you have benign prostate enlargement. Talk to your doctor first if you have symptoms of prostate enlargement.

Taking saw palmetto
You may have to take saw palmetto tincture or capsules for 1–3 months before you see an improvement in your urinary symptoms.

PREVENTION

Reducing urinary problems The following lifestyle changes and remedies may lead to a long-term improvement in urinary symptoms.

- Excess weight puts pressure on your bladder, so try to lose some weight if you need to do so.
- Getting regular exercise can help reduce symptoms caused by an enlarged prostate, while a sedentary lifestyle tends to make them worse.

Erectile dysfunction

Most men experience occasional difficulty in getting or maintaining an erection, often because of stress, fatigue, drinking too much alcohol, or a recent illness. Temporary erectile dysfunction is unlikely to be a cause for concern if you are still able to achieve an erection by masturbating or if you sometimes wake with an erection. Long-term erectile dysfunction can be due to illnesses, such as diabetes and circulatory diseases, or drugs, such as blood pressure medications and antidepressants. It may also be caused by anxiety or depression, or relationship problems. As you get older, it may take longer to get an erection and it may be less firm.

 ## See your doctor first

Make an appointment to see your doctor if:

- You suffer regularly from erectile dysfunction or if you are taking a prescribed drug that may be causing the problem

What you can do yourself

There are several things you can do that may help you overcome temporary erectile dysfunction.

- Don't judge yourself harshly. If you are stressed or tired, for example, because of money concerns, work, or recent illness, tackle the underlying problem.

- If you are in a long-term relationship, talk to your partner. Share your worries, and work together to try to solve the problem. It may help if there is less pressure on you to "perform," so if erection problems are making you nervous about sexual intercourse, try ways of sharing intimacy that reduce sexual anxiety (*see* PRACTICAL TECHNIQUE, right).

- To help relieve anxiety, try practicing deep breathing and muscle relaxation exercises (*see* PRACTICAL TECHNIQUES, pp.20–21).

- Reduce your alcohol intake; even better, avoid it altogether. Drinking too much alcohol can cause difficulty in achieving an erection; recreational drugs can have a similar effect.

- Stop smoking, or at least cut down if you smoke heavily. Young men who smoke double their risk of long-term erectile dysfunction in later life.

PRACTICAL TECHNIQUE

Reducing sexual anxiety Worrying about getting an erection can set up a cycle of "performance anxiety." One of the best ways to reduce anxiety is to take things slowly.

- Take the pressure off. Take turns exploring your partner's body using stroking and massage. You should agree there will be no touching of genitals or breasts at this stage. This will help you both relax.
- After several of these sessions, allow genital and breast stimulation, too, but refrain from intercourse.
- Continue relaxed and leisurely stroking and massage until you begin to get erections again and feel comfortable about proceeding to intercourse.

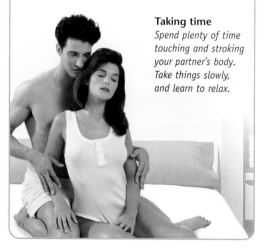

Taking time
Spend plenty of time touching and stroking your partner's body. Take things slowly, and learn to relax.

 ## Seek further medical advice

Arrange to see your doctor if:

- These measures are not helping, or you think erectile dysfunction may have a physical cause

Premature ejaculation

Premature ejaculation, in which a man reaches orgasm and ejaculates with minimum stimulation, just before or shortly after penetration, is a common sexual problem, especially for young men. The problem is mainly due to excitement and/or anxiety and often occurs at the start of a new relationship and resolves itself over time. However, recurrent premature ejaculation can be physically and emotionally frustrating for both partners and may harm a relationship. Stress and depression aggravate the condition; some men become so anxious they have difficulty getting an erection. Rarely, the cause is a prostate or nervous system problem.

 See also **Erectile dysfunction**, opposite page.

What you can do yourself

Because anxiety is a major part of premature ejaculation, talking about the problem with your partner may help to resolve it. There are also several techniques you can try.

● If you are in a long-term relationship, share your feelings with your partner. Discuss the problem calmly and good-humoredly when you are not engaged in sex. Don't blame yourself or feel guilty.

● Some men find wearing a condom dulls sensation sufficiently to delay ejaculation. Some types of condom have a desensitizing lubricant inside that contains a mild topical anesthetic. These may be even more effective. Don't try using anesthetic gel without a condom – it will reduce sensation in your partner, too.

 ● Try using the squeeze technique (*see* PRACTICAL TECHNIQUE, right) to help you control ejaculation.

● Focus your attention on your partner's pleasure during foreplay and delay penetration for as long as possible. If your partner is close to or has reached orgasm before penetration, you will both feel less anxious about premature ejaculation.

● Try experimenting with different sexual positions. Having your partner on top, for example, may be less stimulating and help you delay ejaculation.

● During intercourse, distract yourself by thinking about something totally unrelated and somewhat dull: count backward in threes or think about work.

PRACTICAL TECHNIQUE

The squeeze technique This method of preventing premature ejaculation can be carried out by you or your partner.

● When you feel you're about to ejaculate, use your thumb and forefinger to squeeze the shaft of the penis just below the head, as shown below. This causes your erection to be partially lost, temporarily preventing ejaculation.
● By practicing this technique regularly, you can achieve greater control over ejaculation, and this will boost your sexual confidence. Eventually, you will no longer need to use the technique.

Apply pressure
Use the thumb and forefinger to apply pressure just behind the head of the penis, on the upper and lower sides.

Seek medical advice

Arrange to see your doctor if:

● You continue to experience premature ejaculation after following the advice here

WOMEN'S PROBLEMS

Breast pain and lumpy breasts

Many healthy women experience breast pain (mastalgia) or lumpiness. The symptoms normally affect both breasts and are usually related to hormonal changes during the menstrual cycle. A few days before your menstrual period your breasts may feel swollen, painful, tender, and/or lumpy. These symptoms usually go when the period is over. A more general tendency to breast lumpiness sometimes occurs during adolescence, during pregnancy, or when taking oral contraceptives or hormone therapy. Women who are breast-feeding sometimes develop a red, hot, painful area on one breast due to a buildup of milk or infection (mastitis). Although the majority of breast lumps are not cancer, persistent lumps should always be investigated.

 See also Premenstrual syndrome, p.127.

See your doctor first

Arrange to see your doctor promptly if:

- You find a lump in your breast
- You have lumpiness that persists throughout your menstrual cycle
- You have persistent breast pain that is unrelated to periods, or pain in your armpit
- You think your symptoms may be due to taking oral contraceptives or hormone therapy
- You have symptoms of mastitis

What you can do yourself

Use the following measures to identify and to help alleviate cyclical breast pain or breast lumpiness. (For an attack of mastitis, follow the specific advice on the opposite page.)

- Keep a journal for 2 or 3 menstrual cycles, noting when your breasts become lumpy or sore and when the symptoms pass. This will help you decide if the problem is related to your menstrual cycle.

- Make sure that all your bras fit properly. Try wearing a larger size the week before your period, and/or wear a support bra, such as a sports bra, to reduce breast movement. You may find that wearing a soft bra at night also helps to make you feel more comfortable.

DRUG REMEDIES

Analgesics, such as acetaminophen (*see* p.177) or ibuprofen (*see* p.185), will help relieve discomfort for the few days each month when your breasts are painful. If you are breast-feeding, consult your doctor before you take any medication.

NATURAL REMEDIES

Vitamin B$_6$ supplements (*see* p.189) can help reduce or prevent cyclical breast pain or lumpiness. Usually, you will need to take the supplement for 2–3 months to feel any benefit. Don't exceed the recommended dose, because high doses can be harmful. To boost your intake of B$_6$ from your diet, eat foods such as poultry, eggs, soy, oats, whole-grain bread and cereal, bananas, and nuts.

Foods containing B$_6$
If you prefer not to take vitamin supplements, eat foods that are rich in B$_6$, such as nuts, bananas, and whole-grain bread.

What you can do yourself *continued...*

- Reduce your caffeine intake by cutting down on drinks such as coffee, tea, and cola.

- If you suffer from fluid retention and bloating, cut down on salt the week before your period.

- Increase the amount of carbohydrates in your diet, eat plenty of fresh fruit and vegetables, and avoid fatty food.

- If you are overweight, try losing some weight. Excess fat reserves in your body can affect your hormone levels and contribute to breast pain.

- If tension or stress makes you more susceptible to cyclical breast pain, try practicing some deep breathing and muscle relaxation exercises (*see* PRACTICAL TECHNIQUES, pp.20–21).

 - Take an analgesic on the days when your breasts are painful (*see* DRUG REMEDIES, left).

 - Some women find supplements of vitamin B6 help ease cyclical breast pain and lumpiness (*see* NATURAL REMEDIES, opposite page).

 - Regularly examine your breasts for lumps (*see* PRACTICAL TECHNIQUE, right).

Mastitis

- If you are breast-feeding and you have pain in one breast due to mastitis or milk buildup (engorgement), continue to feed your baby at least every 2 hours from the affected breast, unless your doctor has advised you otherwise. This will keep the milk flowing and keep the breast from getting too full. Alternatively, use a breast pump.

- Make sure your baby is latched on correctly and is sucking properly (*see* PRACTICAL TIPS: BREAST-FEEDING HOLDS FOR SORE NIPPLES, p.126). This will help relieve pressure on the breast.

Seek further medical advice

Arrange to see your doctor if:

- Cyclical breast pain or lumpiness has lasted for more than 2–3 menstrual cycles and is not relieved using self-help measures
- Breast pain is causing you distress and/or is preventing you from carrying out your normal daily activities

PRACTICAL TECHNIQUE

Breast awareness If you examine your breasts once a month, you will know what looks and feels normal for you and find it easier to notice any change. The best time to do this is just after your period, when any hormone-related lumps should have subsided. If you no longer have periods, choose a specific day that will be easy to remember, such as the first day of each month.

1 *Strip to the waist, then stand with your arms by your sides. Look at your breasts in a mirror from the front, then turn and view them from each side to check the outer edges.*

2 *Raise your arms. Look at your breasts from the front and each side. Put your hands on your hips, tense your chest muscles, lean forward, and look again. Each time, check for dimples, puckered skin, changes in size or shape, and changes in the nipples.*

3 *Lie down and put one hand behind your head. Feel the breast on that side, using the flat of your fingers in firm, small, circular movements. Examine the whole breast, including the nipple and armpit. Change hands and repeat the examination for the other breast.*

4 *Note any abnormalities such as tenderness, lumps, swollen veins, or thickened areas. If you discover any changes, consult your doctor.*

Cracked nipples

Many new mothers develop sore, tender nipples during the first few weeks of breast-feeding. One or both nipples may be painful, red, and ridged and may bleed if the skin cracks. Cracked nipples tend to occur when a baby is not positioned properly at the breast and sucks only on the end of the nipple. Women with flat or inverted nipples are susceptible. Sometimes, cracked nipples are due to a yeast infection.

 See also **Feeding problems**, pp.144–145.

 ## See your doctor first

Arrange to see your doctor promptly if:

- Your nipples are red and shiny and have a white deposit on them
- There is a red, tender area on your breast

What you can do yourself

Cracked nipples should heal once you and your baby develop a good breast-feeding technique.

- Check the way you hold your baby at the breast (*see* PRACTICAL TECHNIQUE: SUCCESSFUL BREAST-FEEDING, p.144). Using a new hold may help to reduce pain (*see* PRACTICAL TIPS, right).

- Feed your baby on demand and offer the nipple that is least sore first, when your baby is sucking hardest. Breathe deeply as your baby latches on: a sore nipple is most painful for the first few sucks.

- For flat or inverted nipples, use a lightweight plastic nipple shield to help pull out your nipples.

- Try using a lanolin ointment to help heal deep, painful cracks (*see* DRUG REMEDIES, right).

- After each feeding, wash your nipples with warm water and dry them carefully. Don't use plastic-backed breast pads; they trap moisture. Expose your breasts to the air whenever you can.

- If your nipples are very painful, take acetaminophen (*see* DRUG REMEDIES, right).

 ## Seek further medical advice

Consult your doctor or breast-feeding advisor if:

- Your nipples are not healing within 2–3 days

PRACTICAL TIPS

Breast-feeding holds for sore nipples Holding your baby higher and well supported will reduce painful tugging on a sore nipple.

- Cradle your baby's head high in the crook of the arm with the stomach against your own and the mouth directly facing your nipple. Tuck your baby's arm around your body and keep his or her bottom well supported. Make sure your baby takes the nipple and the darker area around it (areola) into the mouth.
- As an occasional alternative, try the football hold to even out sucking on sore nipples. Using a pillow for support, tuck your baby under your arm with the feet toward your back (like a football player).

Maintaining good support *Hold your baby with his or her front against your body, and support him or her securely.*

DRUG REMEDIES

Lanolin ointment (*see* p.185) formulated for breast-feeding mothers will soothe sore nipples. Rub in a little to protect the skin and help cracks to heal. You don't need to wipe it off before feedings.

Acetaminophen (*see* p.177) will reduce discomfort and help you relax while your baby feeds. Take a dose 30 minutes before a feeding.

Premenstrual syndrome (PMS)

Women with premenstrual syndrome (PMS) are troubled by a variety of symptoms that start about 7 days before a menstrual period and ease when the period begins. You may feel irritable, angry, depressed, or anxious for no particular reason. You may also be absentminded and find it hard to concentrate. Physical symptoms include headache, sleep problems, food cravings, constipation, bloating, weight gain, and breast tenderness or lumpiness. Stress may contribute to the problem.

 See also **Difficulty sleeping**, p.17; **Poor memory**, p.25; **Headache**, p.85; **Bloating and flatulence**, p.108; **Constipation**, p.115; **Breast pain and lumpy breasts**, pp.124–125.

 ## See your doctor first

Arrange to see your doctor if you are not sure that your symptoms are due to PMS.

What you can do yourself

There are a number of remedies that may help PMS. Use them before the first symptoms develop.

● Eat regularly to keep your sugar levels steady and keep you from becoming anxious and irritable. Have plenty of carbohydrates, such as pasta and potatoes, and increase your intake of fruit and vegetables. Avoid sugary snacks; if you are hungry between meals, eat fruit or a whole-wheat cracker.

● Reduce your intake of salt; use herbs and spices to flavor your food instead.

● Drink 6–8 glasses of water a day, and cut down on caffeinated drinks such as coffee. Avoid alcohol in the days before your period.

● Use memory aids such as a notepad or message board to keep track of things you need to do.

● Try to reduce stress (*see* pp.20–21). Postpone big plans and changes, and avoid difficult decisions.

● Go out in the fresh air if possible and take a brisk walk. Get plenty of sleep at night.

 ## Seek further medical advice

Arrange to see your doctor if:

● You still have PMS symptoms after following this advice, or symptoms become worse

 ### PREVENTION

Controlling PMS These longer-term steps may prevent some symptoms of PMS developing and help you cope better with those that remain.

● Keep a journal for 3 months, noting any factors that make PMS symptoms worse, such as particular foods or stress at work, so you can avoid them in the future.

● Try a course of vitamin B$_6$ to help prevent symptoms (*see* NATURAL REMEDIES, below).

● Go for a brisk walk for 20–30 minutes, 5 days a week, or try swimming or practicing yoga regularly.

Yoga exercises
The exercises increase strength and flexibility and will help you relax.

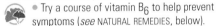 ### NATURAL REMEDIES

Vitamin B$_6$ There is evidence that vitamin B$_6$ (*see* p.189) helps prevent PMS. You may need to take a supplement for 2–3 months before you feel any benefit. Alternatively, boost your diet with foods rich in B$_6$, such as chicken, eggs, bananas, and nuts.

Painful menstrual periods

Many women have a cramping pain in their lower abdomen just before, or at the start of, their monthly period. Some women also have headaches, backache, nausea, and diarrhea. Stress and tension can make symptoms worse. Painful periods most commonly affect younger women and often become less severe with age or after childbirth. They don't usually have a serious underlying cause.

 See also Diarrhea, p.116; Premenstrual syndrome (PMS), p.127.

What you can do yourself

You can usually relieve the symptoms of painful periods using self-help measures.

● To relieve abdominal pain and other aches and pains, take ibuprofen (*see* DRUG REMEDIES, right). You can also soak in a warm bath or apply heat to your abdomen using a heating pad or a hot-water bottle.

● Taking exercise, such as a brisk walk, may bring relief because it stimulates muscles to produce natural painkilling chemicals called endorphins. In the longer term, regular exercise may also help prevent menstrual cramps or reduce their severity.

● Try to avoid stress and tasks that you find physically and/or mentally tiring.

● To reduce anxiety and tension, try practicing some deep breathing and muscle relaxation exercises (*see* PRACTICAL TECHNIQUES, pp.20–21).

● Taking vitamin B6 supplements and/or eating oily fish containing essential fatty acids may help reduce menstrual cramps (*see* NATURAL REMEDIES, right).

 ## Seek medical advice

Arrange to see your doctor if:

● You have bleeding between periods
● Pain continues after your period has finished and/or you have an offensive vaginal discharge
● You wish to discuss taking oral contraceptives, which may help reduce period pain
● The measures given above are not helping to control the pain

DRUG REMEDIES

Ibuprofen (*see* p.185) is an anti-inflammatory drug that helps to reduce cramping and bleeding. If you are prone to menstrual pain, begin taking it before you expect your period to start. If you can't take ibuprofen, use acetaminophen (*see* p.177).

NATURAL REMEDIES

Vitamin B6 supplements (*see* p.189) may help relieve symptoms. Alternatively, eat foods that are rich in the vitamin, such as nuts, soy, and bananas.

Oily fish such as salmon and mackerel contain omega-3 essential fatty acids (*see* p.182), which are thought to affect levels of prostaglandin, a hormone-like substance that can cause menstrual cramps.

Omega-3 source
Try to include oily fish, such as salmon, in your diet about 2–3 times a week.

PREVENTION

Stopping smoking You may be able to prevent or reduce menstrual pain by giving up smoking. This is because smoking has been shown to increase the strength and duration of menstrual cramps.

Menopausal problems

Menopause is a natural change that usually occurs in women between 45 and 55 years, due to falling levels of the female hormone estrogen. At first, your menstrual periods become irregular and light; then they stop. You are considered to be menopausal when you haven't had a period for a year. Some women have no further symptoms, but others have various problems, including hot flashes, night sweats, vaginal dryness, urinary problems, thinning bones, and fatigue.

 See also **Fatigue**, p.15; **Poor bladder control**, p.131; **Painful intercourse**, p.134.

 ### See your doctor first

Make an appointment to see your doctor if you are unsure whether your symptoms are due to menopause, or if you wish to discuss hormone therapy.

What you can do yourself

A few self-help measures may be all you need to control menopausal symptoms.

- If you get hot flashes, dress in layers that you can easily remove. Sleep in a cool room under a light comforter or blanket. Take showers, or warm rather than hot baths. Avoid spicy and hot foods, and cut down on coffee, tea, and alcohol.

 - If you have vaginal dryness and find sex painful, try a lubricating jelly (*see* DRUG REMEDIES, right).

 - Eat calcium-rich foods to help prevent osteoporosis (*see* NATURAL REMEDIES, right). Go out in the sun from time to time; sunlight stimulates vitamin D production, which helps your body absorb calcium.

 - Try including soy products, which contain phyto-estrogens, in your diet (*see* NATURAL REMEDIES, right).

- Drink a lot of water: 6–8 glasses a day.

- If you're feeling tense, try practicing muscle relaxation exercises (*see* PRACTICAL TECHNIQUE, p.21).

- Take regular weight-bearing exercise to relieve stress and strengthen your bones. Brisk walking for about 20–30 minutes a day, 5 days a week, is ideal.

- Avoid smoking – it can worsen symptoms and increase the risk of heart disease and stroke.

 ## DRUG REMEDIES

Lubricating jelly (*see* p.186) will help make sexual intercourse more comfortable. You can either use a gel just before intercourse to lubricate the vagina, or try a longer-acting vaginal moisturizer.

 ## NATURAL REMEDIES

Calcium is found in many foods, including dark green, leafy vegetables such as broccoli; dairy products; and canned fish with edible bones, such as sardines or salmon.

Phytoestrogens (*see* p.188) are natural plant chemicals, found in soy-based foods, that act like estrogen in the body. Eating foods rich in phyto-estrogens, such as soy beans and tofu, may help reduce hot flashes and strengthen bones.

Stir-fried tofu
Rich in phytoestrogens, tofu can be included in many healthy meals.

 ### Seek further medical advice

Arrange to see your doctor if:

- Self-help is not relieving your symptoms
- You develop new symptoms, such as vaginal bleeding, after having had no periods for 1 year

Cystitis

Cystitis is inflammation of the bladder, usually as a result of an infection. If you have an episode of cystitis, you will probably feel a burning pain when you urinate and have the urge to urinate frequently, even when your bladder is empty. The urine may be cloudy and foul smelling, and you may have pain in your lower abdomen. Episodes are sometimes triggered by sexual intercourse. Cystitis is a common condition in women, but is much less common in men and children.

 ## See your doctor first

Make an appointment to see your doctor if:

- You are pregnant
- There is blood in your urine
- You have pain in your back, or in your sides just below your ribs; high fever; or shivering
- Your symptoms are not relieved within 48 hours using the measures below

Men and children with symptoms of cystitis should always see a doctor.

What you can do yourself

Using these simple measures promptly may be enough to clear up a mild episode of cystitis. However, antibiotics may be necessary.

- Drink plenty of fluids to wash away bacteria and keep the urine dilute. This will help make your urine less irritating to the bladder.

- Avoid citrus fruits, tomatoes, spicy foods, caffeine, alcohol, and nicotine. All of these substances can irritate the bladder.

 - Take a cystitis pain relief preparation (*see* DRUG REMEDIES, right) to help relieve the symptoms of cystitis, in conjunction with any treatment provided by your doctor.

 - Hold a covered hot-water bottle over your lower abdomen to relieve any pain, and/or take an analgesic (*see* DRUG REMEDIES, right).

 - Cranberry juice may help to relieve symptoms or even prevent cystitis (*see* NATURAL REMEDIES, right).

- Try to urinate immediately before and after sexual intercourse, to help flush out any bacteria.

 ### DRUG REMEDIES

Cystitis pain relief preparations (*see* p.181) usually contain phenazopyridine to help relieve pain and the burning sensation associated with cystitis, as well as the feeling of needing to urinate urgently.

Analgesics, such as acetaminophen (*see* p.177), can help relieve some of the discomfort of cystitis.

 ### NATURAL REMEDIES

Cranberry juice is a useful treatment that helps to fight infection and may prevent recurrences of cystitis by reducing levels of bacteria in the bladder.

Drinking cranberry juice
Choose a juice with a high proportion of cranberry, and drink 1–2 glasses a day.

 ### PREVENTION

Avoiding recurrences The following measures can help to prevent attacks of cystitis.

- Drink 8 glasses (2–3 quarts) of fluids each day, including 1–2 glasses of cranberry juice.
- Empty your bladder frequently and completely.
- After a bowel movement, wipe from front to back to avoid spreading bacteria.
- Urinate before and after sexual intercourse.
- Wear cotton underwear and avoid tight pants.
- Don't use vaginal deodorants.
- Take showers instead of baths, if possible.

Poor bladder control

Many women suffer from poor bladder control. If you have a condition called stress incontinence, for example, you may leak small amounts of urine when you cough, sneeze, exercise, or lift something heavy. This can be due to weakness in the pelvic floor muscles (which support your bladder, uterus, and rectum) and is common in women who have had children. Other causes of stress incontinence include constipation, bladder infections, hormonal changes after menopause, and some drugs (such as diuretics). Some women have a problem called urge incontinence, which causes sudden urges to urinate or a large leakage without warning. This condition is sometimes due to a disorder that affects the nerves controlling the bladder.

 See also Constipation, p.115; Cystitis, opposite page.

 ## See your doctor first

Make an appointment to see your doctor if:

- You have large leakages of urine
- You are also thirsty and drinking a lot of fluid
- You leak urine without warning, or can't get to the toilet fast enough
- You are taking a prescribed medicine that may be causing poor bladder control

What you can do yourself

There are several steps you can take to improve bladder control if you have stress incontinence, or to supplement treatment from your doctor.

- Drink 6–8 glasses of fluid a day so that your urine doesn't become too concentrated, but don't drink too much in a short time since this may cause leaks.

- Try to lengthen the periods between urinating to gradually improve the capacity of your bladder. Take your time on the toilet so your bladder empties completely. Empty your bladder before going to bed.

- Cut down on tea, coffee, cola, and alcohol; they may cause a sudden and/or uncontrollable urge to urinate. Avoid carbonated drinks, citrus fruits and juices, and spicy foods; they may irritate your bladder.

 - Do Kegel exercises every day (*see* PRACTICAL TECHNIQUE, right).

- If you leak urine during activities such as running or aerobics, insert a tampon just beforehand to help support the bladder. Remove it promptly afterward. Use only as an occasional measure.

 PRACTICAL TECHNIQUE

Kegel exercises can be done anywhere, sitting or standing. It may take up to 12 weeks for you to benefit, and you will need to keep doing them to prevent symptoms from recurring.

- Tighten and release your pelvic floor muscles: these are the muscles you use to stop urinating midstream.
- Squeeze the muscles, hold for a few seconds, then relax slowly. Repeat several times. Gradually build up to 10 squeezes, taking 10 seconds for each and resting for about 4 seconds between squeezes.
- Do the exercises regularly throughout every day until they become second nature.

 PREVENTION

Bladder care Over time, these measures will reduce pressure and irritation affecting your bladder.

- Try to lose any excess weight.
- Eat plenty of fiber to prevent constipation.
- Stop smoking. Nicotine irritates the bladder, and smoke can make you cough and strain your muscles.

 ## Seek further medical advice

Arrange to see your doctor if:

- Incontinence gets worse
- You see little or no improvement in your bladder control after 4–6 weeks
- You develop other symptoms

Vaginal discharge

It is normal for a woman to have some discharge from the vagina. This is usually clear or white, the amount and consistency varying at different times in the menstrual cycle, during pregnancy, and in response to sexual arousal. However, a profuse discharge or one that has an unusual consistency or smell is usually a sign of infection. The most common cause is a yeast infection that produces a discharge like cottage cheese, irritation in or around your vagina, and, sometimes, a burning sensation when you pass urine. This is not usually sexually transmitted. It is caused by factors that encourage overgrowth of yeast, such as taking antibiotics, wearing tight-fitting clothes, and using vaginal douches and deodorants. Some types of vaginal discharge are a symptom of a sexually transmitted infection and need treatment from a doctor.

 ## See your doctor first

Make an appointment to see your doctor if you think you may have a sexually transmitted infection and/or:

- The discharge is bloodstained, greenish yellow, or foul smelling
- You have other symptoms, such as fever and lower abdominal pain
- You have recurrent abnormal discharges
- You are pregnant

What you can do yourself

If you are sure that you have a yeast infection, you can usually treat it yourself. Start the treatment as soon as you notice symptoms.

 - Use an antifungal suppository or cream for a yeast infection (*see* DRUG REMEDIES, right).

 - To relieve itchiness and discomfort, try adding some baking soda to a bath (*see* NATURAL REMEDIES, right).

 - For a mild yeast infection, applying yogurt to your vulva and vagina may help (*see* NATURAL REMEDIES, right). This has a soothing effect.

 ## Seek further medical advice

Arrange to see your doctor if:

- The infection does not clear up in 2–3 days using the treatment above or from your doctor

 ### DRUG REMEDIES

Antifungal drugs (*see* p.178) come in two types. You can take a short course of clotrimazole or miconazole suppositories or cream. These should be introduced into the vagina while you are lying down, so the drug stays in place. Use them at bedtime so that they work overnight.

 ### NATURAL REMEDIES

Baking soda (*see* p.179) can help to soothe soreness and irritation. Add 2 tablespoonfuls to a lukewarm, shallow bath.

Yogurt with active cultures contains bacteria that help fight the infection. To insert yogurt into your vagina, put some in the top of a tampon applicator, then insert the tampon into the vagina. Remove it an hour later.

Using yogurt
Apply it to your vulva and inside your vagina.

 ### PREVENTION

Avoiding attacks If you often have yeast infections, the following may help prevent recurrences.

- Don't use pantyhose, synthetic panties, or panty liners. Use only sanitary pads during periods. If you use tampons, change them at least every 4 hours.
- Use only water and unperfumed soap on your vulva.

Genital irritation

Itching inside the vagina or around the vulva (the folds of skin outside the vagina) may be uncomfortable and embarrassing during the day and make it difficult for you to sleep at night. The area may be dry, red, and swollen and you may have a stinging sensation when you urinate and/or discomfort during sex. Symptoms are usually worse in hot weather. Genital irritation is often a reaction to soaps and perfumes in toiletries, but it can also be due to an infection, another skin condition, or to not drying yourself properly after using the toilet.

 See also **Vaginal discharge**, opposite page; **Painful intercourse**, p.134.

 ## See your doctor first

Make an appointment to see your doctor if:

- You have a discharge, or painful urination
- You have itching elsewhere and/or have a skin condition such as eczema or psoriasis
- You are losing weight without trying and/or are drinking or urinating more than usual
- You have black specks in your pubic hair

What you can do yourself

Try the following home treatments to help relieve itching and reduce inflammation.

- Use a cold compress. Wrap a pack of frozen peas or crushed ice in a wet towel, or soak a washcloth in cold water, then wring it out. Apply it gently to your vulva, as often as needed. You could also sit in a shallow, cool or lukewarm bath for 10–15 minutes.

 - Try a moisturizing cream or ointment to soothe the inflamed skin (*see* DRUG REMEDIES, right).

 - Take a sedative antihistamine to reduce irritation and help you sleep (*see* DRUG REMEDIES, right).

 - Use a vaginal lubricant if your vagina feels dry or sore during sex (*see* DRUG REMEDIES, right).

- Resist the urge to scratch your vulva. In bed, wear a nightgown without underwear to let the air circulate around your genital area.

 ## Seek further medical advice

Arrange to see your doctor if:

- Irritation persists for more than 3–4 days

 ## DRUG REMEDIES

Moisturizers (*see* p.187), such as water-based cream and emulsifying ointment, soothe irritated skin. Apply a moisturizer to your vulva about 3 times a day, and use it as a substitute for soap when washing.

Antihistamines (*see* p.178) relieve itching. A sedative antihistamine, taken at bedtime, will also make it easier for you to sleep.

Vaginal lubricants (*see* LUBRICATING JELLY, p.186) will help to make sexual intercourse more comfortable. Either use a gel just before intercourse or try a longer-acting vaginal moisturizer.

 ## PREVENTION

Avoiding irritation You can help prevent genital irritation by avoiding possible triggers and being extra careful with personal hygiene.

- Don't use perfumed soaps, bubble baths, vaginal deodorants, or douches. Wash your genital area once or twice a day with plain warm water or an unperfumed soap. Pat yourself dry with a soft towel, or use a hair dryer on a cool setting for a few seconds.
- Put your laundry through an extra rinse and don't use fabric softeners.
- Wipe yourself from front to back after a bowel movement and dry yourself thoroughly after urinating. Use soft, unbleached, uncolored toilet paper.
- Ask your partner to switch to nonlatex condoms or those without spermicide. Don't use deodorized sanitary pads or panty liners.
- Wear comfortable cotton underwear, and change it daily. Choose pantyhose with a cotton gusset, or stockings. Don't wear tight-fitting jeans.
- Take off your swimsuit promptly after swimming.

Painful intercourse

Many women experience painful sexual intercourse from time to time. Sometimes, the problem is a physical one: for example, sex is often uncomfortable after childbirth, particularly if you had stitches or a tear, or after menopause when the vagina is less well lubricated. Vaginal infections and irritations, or simply being constipated, can also play a part. Vaginal dryness due to lack of arousal is often a factor in painful intercourse; in extreme cases, a woman may experience spasms in her vaginal muscles that make penetration difficult or even impossible. Physical symptoms such as these are often due to underlying psychological factors such as anxiety, guilt, or previous experience of painful intercourse.

 ## See your doctor first

Make an appointment to see your doctor if:

- You have deep pelvic pain during intercourse
- Vaginal spasms and/or emotional problems may be contributing to painful intercourse

What you can do yourself

If you find intercourse painful, try to identify the cause and take the following steps as appropriate.

- Try using a lubricating jelly (*see* DRUG REMEDIES, right) if you suffer from vaginal dryness.

- If a certain sexual position causes pain, try another one. Some women like to be on top, so that they can control penetration.

- If you think that vaginal dryness might be due to lack of arousal, talk things through with your partner. Make sure you spend enough time on foreplay. Caressing each other without progressing to full intercourse from time to time will take the pressure off and help you both relax.

- Painful intercourse can make you anxious and more likely to tighten up the next time you try to have sex. You may be able to break this vicious circle by spending more time on foreplay as above, soaking in a warm bath, having a glass of wine, and practicing muscle relaxation exercises (*see* PRACTICAL TECHNIQUE, p.21) before you have sex.

- Don't use douches or perfumed toiletries in case they cause vaginal discomfort and irritation.

- If you use tampons, check you have not forgotten to remove one at the end of your last period.

DRUG REMEDIES

Lubricating jelly (*see* p.186) Apply a water-soluble jelly to your vagina before you have sexual intercourse. Alternatively, use a longer-lasting vaginal moisturizer that replenishes moisture over several days.

Using lubricants
Long-acting moisturizers are supplied with an applicator, which is inserted into the vagina. Apply jelly with an applicator or with your fingers.

 ## Seek further medical advice

Arrange to see your doctor if:

- The pain continues despite treating the cause and using self-help measures
- You develop other symptoms, such as bleeding from the vagina after intercourse

CHILDREN'S PROBLEMS

Fever (children)

A child with a fever has a temperature raised persistently above 98.6°F (37°C). Children develop a fever more easily than adults. Causes may include a minor illness, such as a cold, ear infection, or chickenpox, or simply being overdressed. A feverish child looks bright-eyed and flushed, and the forehead and neck feel hot. Some children feel tired, shiver, and have a headache.

 See also **Febrile seizures**, p.167.

WARNING

Seek immediate medical help if:
● Your child has a headache and stiff neck, is sensitive to bright light, and/or develops a rash (*see* p.150)
● He or she is drowsy, is breathing fast, or has had a seizure

See your doctor first

Arrange to see your doctor promptly if your child also has earache, a rash, or a sore throat.

What you can do yourself

Use the self-help treatments described below to make a feverish child more comfortable.

● Make sure your child gets plenty of rest, although he or she does not need to stay in bed.

 ● Give an analgesic such as acetaminophen or ibuprofen to reduce fever (*see* DRUG REMEDIES, right) and give your child plenty of cool drinks.

 ● You can get a good idea of your child's temperature by feeling his or her forehead or the back of the neck. If you need an accurate result, use a thermometer (*see* PRACTICAL TECHNIQUE, right).

● Dress your child in light clothing. Don't swaddle the child in blankets, even if he or she has chills. Make sure the room is comfortable and not too hot.

Seek further medical advice

Arrange to see your doctor if:
● Your child does not improve within 24 hours
● His or her temperature continues to rise
● He or she develops new symptoms

DRUG REMEDIES

Analgesics include acetaminophen (*see* p.177), available as drops, liquid medicine, or chewable tablets, or ibuprofen (*see* p.185), available as drops. Make sure you ask your pharmacist to recommend an appropriate product for your child. If your child spits the medicine out, try using an oral syringe (available from your pharmacist).

PRACTICAL TECHNIQUE

Taking a child's temperature Use an easy-to-read digital thermometer, which is placed in your child's mouth or armpit, or an aural sensor thermometer, the tip of which is inserted into the ear. Take a reading every 2–3 hours. Forehead temperature strips are unreliable, and mercury thermometers are no longer recommended.

Aural thermometer
Gently insert the tip for a few seconds. Remove the thermometer to read the display.

Diarrhea and vomiting (children)

Diarrhea and vomiting in a child is often due to gastroenteritis, an infection that can be picked up through contact with infected people or from contaminated food or water. Your child may also have abdominal pains, fever, and a headache. Emotional stress or excitement can cause an upset stomach in some children, as can reactions to food or drink, particularly large amounts of fruit or sugar. Children sometimes develop toddler's diarrhea – watery stools in which bits of food can be seen – due to not digesting food properly. This usually clears up by the age of 3. A child with an illness that causes a fever or cough may vomit without diarrhea.

 See also **Food intolerance**, p.113; **Food poisoning**, p.114.

 ## See your doctor first

Make an appointment to see your doctor if:

- There is blood in your child's stools or vomit
- Your child has sunken eyes, a dry mouth and tongue, has not urinated for more than 6 hours, or is abnormally drowsy
- Your child gets repeated bouts of diarrhea

What you can do yourself

If your child has vomiting and diarrhea the main risk is dehydration, so you need to replace lost fluids.

 - Make sure your child has plenty to drink. If he or she is still vomiting, give frequent sips of water. You can use an oral rehydration solution to replace lost fluids and salts (*see* DRUG REMEDIES, right).

- When your child feels ready to eat again, start by offering small amounts of bland foods, then gradually return to a normal diet.

 - Give your child acetaminophen to ease a fever or stomachache (*see* DRUG REMEDIES, right), but don't give over-the-counter antidiarrheal medicines.

 ## Seek further medical advice

Arrange to see your doctor if:

- Your child has abdominal pain for more than 3 hours; vomiting has not stopped after 12 hours; or diarrhea has not stopped after 24 hours
- Your child is refusing drinks

 ### DRUG REMEDIES

Oral rehydration solutions (*see* p.188) replace water, salts, and sugars lost from diarrhea and/or vomiting and prevent dehydration. They are available as ready-to-use bottled solutions in different flavors.

Acetaminophen (*see* p.177) will help to relieve fever and pain due to gastroenteritis.

 Rehydration drink
Offer oral rehydration solution instead of, or in addition to, the child's regular drinks.

 ### PREVENTION

Avoiding infection Be scrupulous about hygiene to prevent infection with gastroenteritis or, if your child already has the infection, to stop it from being passed to other family members.

- Wash your hands thoroughly with soap and water before and after handling or feeding your child; before handling food or eating; and after using the toilet. Make sure other family members do the same.
- Use separate towels and washcloths for your child if he or she has an infection.
- Clean the toilet regularly, including the seat and handle, with bleach or disinfectant.
- Make sure your child washes his or her hands after playing outdoors or handling pets.

Pinworms

Pinworms most often affect children. You may notice the tiny worms, like threads of cotton, in your child's stools, but usually the first sign is itching around the anus (and vulva in girls) at night when the worms lay eggs. If your child scratches, the area may become sore and your child may pick up eggs on his or her fingers and reingest them or pass them to others. If many worms are present, your child may have a stomachache.

 See also Itchy anus, p.118.

 ## See your doctor first

Make an appointment to see your doctor if you are not sure that your child has a pinworm infestation, or if a child under 2 years has pinworms.

What you can do yourself

Pinworm infestation is usually easy to treat at home with medicine and hygiene measures.

- Give your child a pinworm treatment to kill the worms (*see* DRUG REMEDIES, right). Treat all other family members at the same time, even if they don't have symptoms.

- Have your child wear underpants at night to help prevent scratching.

- Bathe your child, or wash around his or her anus, every morning to remove any worm eggs that have been laid during the night.

- Ensure your child takes particular care with hygiene (*see* PRACTICAL TIPS, right).

- You don't need to keep your child out of school or separated from friends, but do remind him or her to be especially careful about personal hygiene while away from home.

- You don't need to treat pets such as cats and dogs: they don't carry pinworms.

 ## Seek further medical advice

Arrange to see your doctor if:

- Your child continues to have symptoms after about 2–3 weeks despite treatment

 ### DRUG REMEDIES

Pinworm treatments (*see* p.188) include the worm-paralyzing drug pyrantel, which is the usual treatment for anyone over 2 years old. It is available as a capsule or as a liquid to be taken by mouth. A single dose should be effective, although a second dose after 2–3 weeks is sometimes required. Make an appointment to see your doctor if a child under the age of 2 has pinworms. These drugs affect the worms but not their eggs, so be very careful about hygiene for at least 2 weeks after administering treatment.

CAUTION: If you are pregnant or breast-feeding, consult your doctor before using these treatments.

 ### PRACTICAL TIPS

Essential hygiene Be scrupulous about hygiene to break the worm's lifecycle, and to prevent reinfestation and spread to other people.

- Ensure your child washes his or her hands before eating or handling food, and after using the toilet. Keep nails short and discourage finger-sucking and nail-biting.
- Eggs can survive for 2 weeks on items such as bedding and towels, so change these daily. Don't shake them out because you may spread the eggs. Wash items in hot water and dry them in a tumble-dryer. Give your child a washcloth and towel for his or her own use.

Treating nails
Scrub under the nails to remove any eggs that may be lodged there.

Croup

Croup is a viral infection normally affecting children between 3 months and 3 years old. It usually begins with symptoms such as a runny nose, sneezing, and fever. After a day or two, the child develops a barking cough, like a sea lion, and a hoarse voice. Attacks of croup often occur in the early hours of the morning, and if severe, the child makes a whistling noise (stridor) when breathing in. Most children recover in a couple of days, but the cough may take several days longer to clear up.

> ## WARNING
> Seek immediate medical help if:
> ● Your child's breathing is noisy or he or she is having difficulty breathing, speaking, or swallowing
> ● Your child is drooling, or his or her lips or mouth look blue

✚ See your doctor first

Arrange to see your doctor promptly if you think your child has croup, to confirm the diagnosis and get advice on treatment.

What you can do yourself

An attack of croup can be frightening for you and your child. Act quickly to relieve the symptoms.

● Humidify the air in your bathroom and sit there with your child until his or her breathing eases (*see* PRACTICAL TECHNIQUE, right).

● When your child is in bed, increase the humidity in the room by using a humidifier, or place a bowl of water or a wet towel beside a radiator. If you are able to, sleep in the same room as your child so you can keep an eye on his or her breathing.

● Give acetaminophen to bring down a fever (*see* DRUG REMEDIES, right). Don't give cough medicines.

● Encourage your child to rest and take frequent warm drinks during the day.

● Sitting upright will make it easier for your child to breathe. Sit a baby with croup in a baby seat.

✚ Seek further medical advice

Arrange to see your doctor urgently if:

● Your child is still distressed after you have taken steps to treat an attack of croup
● Your child has not recovered from croup after 2 or 3 days of treatment

PRACTICAL TECHNIQUE

Humidifying the air To ease your child's breathing, you will need to sit together in a steamy atmosphere in the bathroom for about 20 minutes. You may want to take something such as a story or picture book into the bathroom to distract your child.

● Close the bathroom door, run the hot faucet into the bath or run the shower, and let the room steam up.
● Sit with your child seated on your knee, supporting his or her back. Be careful to keep the child clear of the hot water.
● Let your child breathe in the moist air for 15–20 minutes, until his or her breathing gets easier. If this does not relieve symptoms, get immediate medical help.

Breathing steam
Keep your child sitting upright and encourage him or her to take slow, deep breaths.

DRUG REMEDIES

Analgesics such as acetaminophen (*see* p.177) and ibuprofen (*see* p.185) can help to reduce fever. Make sure you ask your pharmacist to recommend an appropriate product for your child.

Bedwetting

Although most children become reliably dry at night between the ages of 3 and 7, bedwetting (enuresis) is a common problem for young children. Around 1 in 6 still wet the bed at 5 years; around 1 in 20 are still wetting at age 10. Your child may need treatment if he or she continues after age 7, or starts again after 6 months or more of dry nights. If your child wets the bed regularly, it is most likely to be because he or she has not yet learned bladder control; this will improve in time. Bedwetting is rarely caused by a physical or psychological problem, although a child who has been dry at night may have lapses due to a bladder infection or an emotional upset such as bullying; constipation may also be a contributory factor. Bedwetting tends to run in families.

 ## See your doctor first

Make an appointment to see your doctor if:

- You are concerned about bedwetting, especially if your child is over 7 years old or has previously been dry at night
- Your child has a fever and a burning feeling when urinating, and needs to frequently
- You think your child may be constipated

What you can do yourself

Most children grow out of bedwetting eventually, but in the meantime, try the following steps.

- Never punish your child for bedwetting. Explain to the child that the problem is not his or her fault.

- Don't restrict fluids, but ask your child not to drink anything within 2 or 3 hours of bedtime. Avoid giving chocolate or cola in the early evening.

- Put your child to bed earlier. Make sure he or she uses the toilet before bed. Most bedwetting occurs in the first third of the night, so try waking your child to urinate before you go to bed.

- Don't put your child in diapers at night, because he or she may not then recognize the need to get up and go to the toilet. Instead, use a waterproof-backed oversheet or plastic mattress cover.

- Try linking your child's progress to rewards. For example, take a jar and give the child a marble to drop in it for every dry night. Offer a reward for a certain number of marbles. Ignore any relapses.

 - If the above measures have not worked, you could try a pad and buzzer alarm system (*see* PRACTICAL TECHNIQUE, right).

 ## PRACTICAL TECHNIQUE

Pad and buzzer alarm systems

These systems are sometimes advised for children over 7 years who regularly wet the bed, but they should be used only as a last resort and preferably under medical supervision. They have a moisture-detecting pad which is placed under the bottom sheet, and a buzzer beside the bed. As soon as a child starts to urinate the buzzer sounds, waking the child so he or she can go to the toilet. Over a few months, the child becomes conditioned to wake before the buzzer sounds and becomes dry at night.

Positioning the pad
The pad is placed under the bottom sheet where the child's hips will lie.

Moisture-detection pad

Buzzer

 ## Seek further medical advice

Arrange to see your doctor if:

- Your child's bedwetting persists despite using the measures described above

Earache (children)

Earache is a common childhood complaint often caused by an infection in the middle ear or the outer ear (swimmer's ear). A buildup of fluid behind the eardrum after a cold or a foreign object pushed into the ear can also cause earache. Sometimes the pain is referred from a sore throat or tooth problem. A young child may not be able to say what is wrong but may pull at one ear; have reduced hearing; be distressed; and be feverish if there is an infection. A discharge from the ear may indicate that the eardrum has burst.

 See also Swimmer's ear, p.65; Popping ears, p.66; Foreign object in the ear, p.68.

 ## See your doctor first

Make an appointment to see your doctor if your child has earache to confirm the diagnosis and be advised on treatment.

What you can do yourself

While following your doctor's advice, there are several measures that you can take to relieve your child's earache. The problem can be very upsetting, especially for young children, so you need to calm your child and distract him or her from the pain.

● Sit your child upright, resting on pillows, as this position may help reduce pressure in the middle ear. Your child will probably sleep better propped up on pillows in bed.

 ● Holding a warm towel or well-covered hot-water bottle against the affected ear can help to soothe the pain (*see* PRACTICAL TIP, right).

 ● Give your child an analgesic if the earache is causing distress (*see* DRUG REMEDIES, right).

● If your child's eardrum bursts, gently wipe away the discharge, keep the ear dry, and have it checked by the doctor.

● Don't poke cotton swabs into your child's ear to try to clean it, or insert eardrops or oil unless advised to do so by your doctor.

● Distract your child by reading stories or by playing favorite games.

● Keep your child away from tobacco smoke.

 ### PRACTICAL TIP

Applying warmth Gentle heat can help to relieve an earache. Use a well-wrapped hot-water bottle or heat a towel on a radiator or iron it. Check that it is not too hot, then hold it against the affected ear. For a baby, hold a warm, soft cloth over the ear.

Heat treatment
Resting the painful ear on a covered hot-water bottle for about 20 minutes can soothe earache.

 ### DRUG REMEDIES

Analgesics will help to bring down a fever and reduce the pain of earache. Acetaminophen (*see* p.177) is available as liquid medicine or chewable pills, and ibuprofen (*see* p.185) is available as liquid medicine. Make sure you ask your pharmacist to recommend an appropriate product for your child.

 ## Seek further medical advice

Arrange for your child to see your doctor if:

● The earache becomes more severe, or your child is not beginning to feel better after 1–2 days of using treatment from your doctor

● You are concerned that your child's hearing has not returned to normal following treatment

Temper tantrums

Most parents of young children have some experience of temper tantrums. When a child feels frustrated, tired, hungry, or overstimulated he or she may rage, cry, scream, and stamp, kicking and hitting anyone or anything close by. Some children vomit, or more rarely, hold their breath to the point of fainting. Tantrums start some time after 1 year, reach a peak between 2 and 3, and usually stop by 4 years. They are part of normal development, but avoiding triggers (such as the child being overtired) will make them less frequent.

See your doctor first

Make an appointment to see your doctor if:

- Your child is having breath-holding attacks
- Your child hurts him- or herself or others during temper tantrums

What you can do yourself

During a tantrum, use the following tips to calm the situation and cope with it constructively.

- At the first signs of a tantrum, try to find and deal with the cause. For example, offer a snack if you suspect your child is hungry, or read a story if he or she seems exhausted but too agitated to sleep. Give the child your undivided attention if possible.

- Even if there is no obvious cause for a tantrum, don't get angry. Shouting and hitting will frighten your child and make the behavior worse. Show that you still love your child in spite of the tantrum.

- During a full-blown tantrum, it may be hard to get through to your child. As long as the child is in a safe place and not harming him- or herself or others, it may be better to let the tantrum run its course. Stay where your child can see you.

- If a tantrum happens in a public place, ignore the reaction of other people and try to remove or deal with your child calmly and good-humoredly.

- Don't give in to unreasonable demands or buy your way out of trouble with treats. This will make it more difficult to deal with the next tantrum.

- Breath-holding is usually harmless. During an attack, lay your child flat on the ground. If the child passes out, stay calm; he or she will quickly regain consciousness. If there is any delay or you are concerned, however, seek immediate medical help.

PREVENTION

Avoiding triggers for tantrums

If your child is prone to temper tantrums, it helps to identify situations and frustrations that trigger them. Avoiding them may prevent some tantrums or at least make them milder and less distressing.

- Don't ignore your child. If you are engrossed in other activities, such as speaking on the phone or trying to finish some work, take a break.
- Have reasonable expectations. Notice and reward positive behavior in your child and ignore minor negative behavior. Don't fight over trivial matters.
- Save a firm "no" for things that are important, such as safety issues or behavior that causes potential harm to the child or to others.
- Give your child some control by offering choices instead of instructions. Limit the choices to a simple "either/or" for a young child, such as "Would you like to wear your shoes or your sandals?" or "Would you like to go to the park or play in the garden?"
- Try to keep to regular meals, sleep, and playtimes to prevent your child from becoming hungry or overtired. If there is a change in the daily schedule, prepare your child by explaining as much as can be understood and by ensuring that the child has a favorite item such as a toy or book.
- Young children are often frustrated because they cannot express themselves. Talk to, listen to, and watch your child carefully so you are tuned in to his or her needs, likes, and dislikes.

Seek further medical advice

Arrange to see your doctor if:

- You cannot cope with your child's tantrums
- Tantrums and breath-holding attacks continue after the age of 4

PROBLEMS IN BABIES

Fever (babies)

A baby with a fever has a temperature that is raised persistently above 98.6°F (37°C). He or she may look flushed, and the forehead, back of the neck, and body will feel hot, although the hands and feet may be cold. The baby may be irritable and refuse feedings. Fever is often due to an infection such as a cold, or to being too hot or overdressed. Mild fever after immunizations is also common.

 See also Febrile seizures, p.167.

WARNING
Seek immediate medical help if:
- Your baby's breathing is fast or labored, or he or she is drowsy
- Your baby has had a convulsion
- Your baby has a red rash that does not fade when pressed (*see* p.150)

See your doctor first

Arrange to see your doctor promptly if:

- Your baby is under 6 months old
- An older baby is not feeding and/or has vomiting and diarrhea or a rash, or you are in any way concerned about your baby

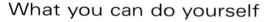

What you can do yourself

You should be able to reduce a fever using the following steps, although a mild fever can often be left to run its course if your baby is otherwise well.

- Undress your baby down to a diaper and undershirt to cool him or her down. Don't overdress your baby or swaddle him or her in blankets – babies can overheat if dressed or covered too warmly.

- Take your baby's temperature (*see* PRACTICAL TECHNIQUE: TAKING A CHILD'S TEMPERATURE, p.135).

 - Give an analgesic to reduce your baby's temperature (*see* DRUG REMEDIES, right).

- Give your baby cooled, boiled water in a bottle in between bottle feedings. If you are breast-feeding, try to increase the length or frequency of feedings.

- Make sure your baby's room is at a comfortable temperature. Use an electric fan if the room is hot.

- Sponging or bathing with lukewarm water is not recommended since it may worsen a fever.

DRUG REMEDIES

Analgesics such as acetaminophen and ibuprofen can be given in liquid form to reduce a baby's fever. If your baby spits the medicine out, try using a syringe (available from your pharmacist) to introduce it slowly, but don't squirt it into the back of the mouth since it may cause choking. Don't give acetaminophen to babies under 2 years of age or ibuprofen to babies under 6 months, except on a doctor's advice.

Medicine syringe
Gently squirt the medicine into the inside of your baby's cheek.

Seek further medical advice

Arrange to see your doctor if:

- Your baby is not getting better within 24 hours, or his or her temperature continues to rise despite the measures described above
- Your baby develops new symptoms

Diarrhea and vomiting (babies)

Many babies normally have semiliquid feces, and regurgitate small amounts of milk after a feeding, but diarrhea and vomiting are more serious. An affected baby passes runny feces more frequently than normal and may vomit whole feedings. The most common cause of prolonged diarrhea and vomiting is gastroenteritis (inflammation of the stomach and intestines), which mainly affects bottle-fed babies. Although it usually clears up quickly, there is a risk of your baby becoming dehydrated.

WARNING

Seek immediate medical help if:
- Your baby is under 3 months old
- Your baby has blood- or green-stained vomit; bloody or tarry stools; sunken eyes; dry mouth and tongue; dry diapers; or is drowsy

 See also **Feeding problems**, pp.144–145.

What you can do yourself

There are several steps you can take to relieve mild diarrhea and vomiting. The main risk is dehydration, so it is important to replace lost fluids.

 ● If you are breast-feeding, don't stop. Offer your baby more frequent feedings. If diarrhea worsens, give your baby an oral rehydration preparation after each feeding (*see* DRUG REMEDIES, right).

 ● If bottle-feeding, continue full-strength feedings but give smaller amounts more frequently. Offer an oral rehydration solution (*see* DRUG REMEDIES, right) instead of feedings if your baby refuses formula, or as well as feedings if diarrhea worsens. Increase fluids gradually; too much may encourage vomiting.

● If your baby is taking solids, keep to a normal diet if he or she feels like eating. If your baby has no appetite or continues to vomit, the most important thing is to keep giving fluids. When your baby feels like eating again, offer small amounts of bland foods such as apple purée, mashed banana, and mashed potatoes. Gradually build up the quantities and variety as your baby improves, returning to a normal diet as soon as he or she can tolerate it.

 ## Seek further medical advice

Arrange to see your doctor if:

- Your baby's condition is getting worse
- Your baby is not taking fluids
- He or she has had diarrhea for 24 hours, or has been vomiting for longer than 3 hours

DRUG REMEDIES

Oral rehydration solutions (see p.188), available from your pharmacist, are designed to replace water, sugar, and salts lost from diarrhea and vomiting and to prevent dehydration. They are available as ready-to-use bottled solutions and come in several different flavors. Use the solution within 48 hours of opening.

Rehydration
Give your baby rehydration solutions in a bottle to help prevent dehydration.

PREVENTION

Be scrupulous about hygiene
This will help prevent your baby from getting gastroenteritis or, if he or she has the infection, will stop it from being passed to other family members.

- Wash your hands thoroughly with soap and water before and after handling or feeding your baby; before handling food or eating; and after using the toilet. Make sure everyone in the family does the same.
- Use separate towels and washcloths for your baby if he or she has an infection.
- Wash your baby's hands after he or she has been playing outdoors or handling pets.

Feeding problems

Most feeding problems in babies occur in the early months. Some newborns need practice at latching on to the breast, while bottle-fed babies may have trouble with different sizes of nipples and types of formula. Babies who are not getting enough milk are often excessively sleepy and slow to gain weight, while those who are overfed gain weight too quickly. Many breast-fed and bottle-fed babies effortlessly spit up small amounts of milk after a feeding; this is not a cause for concern. Some, however, regurgitate larger amounts of feeding and may wheeze. This condition, called reflux, may last for up to a year and is due to a weak muscle at the entrance to the stomach. It is most common in premature babies or those whose muscle tone is poor. A baby who feeds well but wakes screaming between feedings may have an allergy to milk.

 See also Cracked nipples, p.126; **Colic**, p.148.

 ## See your doctor first

Make an appointment to see your doctor if:

- Your baby can't feed or won't feed
- Your baby has been feeding well, but has developed problems
- Your baby regurgitates large volumes of milk and/or there is blood in the vomit
- Your baby fails to gain or loses weight

What you can do yourself

Most feeding problems resolve themselves over time, but using the following tips will help. You can be sure that your newborn baby is feeding well if he or she produces 6 or more wet diapers a day, sleeps well, and gains weight at the predicted rate.

- Make sure your newborn baby feeds properly at least 6 times in 24 hours. Don't assume a sleepy baby is "content"; wake your baby for feedings if he or she is sleeping for more than 4 hours.

- Babies who gain weight too fast are usually bottle-fed. Ask your doctor for advice about how to regulate feeding.

- If your baby tends to spit up milk after a feeding, change the diaper beforehand so that you don't have to disturb your baby too much after he or she has fed. Pause and burp your baby at intervals during the feeding, and hold him or her upright on your lap afterward to allow gas to come up naturally. If you are bottle-feeding, try using a bottle and nipple specifically designed to reduce gas.

PRACTICAL TECHNIQUE

Successful breast-feeding It may take a little practice for both you and your baby to get breast-feeding right. These simple steps will help.

- Hold your baby with the head cradled in the crook of your arm, the bottom well supported and the arm tucked around your body. Whenever possible, have skin to skin contact with your baby during feedings.
- Stroke your baby's cheek with a finger or your nipple so that the mouth opens wide and your baby turns toward the nipple. Expressing a little milk onto the nipple will help encourage your baby.
- Aiming your nipple at the roof of the baby's mouth, make sure the nipple and as much of the areola around it as possible is taken into the mouth. When the baby closes his or her mouth it will form a tight seal.
- If your baby sucks only on the end of the nipple, he or she will not be getting milk and your nipple may become sore. Ease the baby off the breast by gently inserting a finger into the corner of the mouth and reposition him or her to try again.

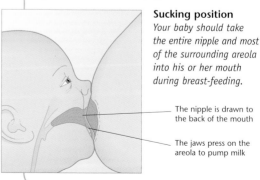

Sucking position
Your baby should take the entire nipple and most of the surrounding areola into his or her mouth during breast-feeding.

The nipple is drawn to the back of the mouth

The jaws press on the areola to pump milk

What you can do yourself *continued...*

- A baby who has been diagnosed with reflux needs a special feeding regimen until he or she grows out of the condition (*see* PRACTICAL TIPS, right).

Breast-feeding

- If you have not breast-fed before, there are several tips that will help get you off to a good start (*see* PRACTICAL TECHNIQUE, left). Make sure you have help from someone who has had experience in breast-feeding.

- Your baby may find it hard to latch on if your breasts are engorged or very full. Expressing a little milk before he or she begins to feed will soften the breast. This will also help if your baby chokes because your milk flows too fast.

- Until your baby has learned to breast-feed properly, don't use pacifiers or bottles.

- Occasionally expressing milk by hand or using a breast pump between feedings will help empty the breast and stimulate a good supply of milk. This also helps draw out a flat or inverted nipple, as does wearing a nipple shield.

- Make sure you eat an extra 500 calories a day and rest whenever you can to maintain a good milk supply for your baby.

- If your baby is unsettled and wakes screaming between feedings, try excluding dairy products from your diet for a week to see if the problem is due to an allergic reaction to them. If symptoms improve, continue these measures.

Bottle-feeding

- If your baby is feeding too slowly, try a nipple with a larger hole. Conversely, a baby who gulps and feeds too fast may need a nipple with a smaller hole.

- Try changing to a different milk formula if your baby is consistently unsettled or unhappy after feeding. If he or she wakes screaming between feedings, try a hypoallergenic formula for a week to see if the problem is due to milk allergy. If symptoms improve, continue these measures.

- If your baby has diarrhea and vomiting (*see* p.143), be careful about washing your hands before a feeding and be meticulous about sterilizing bottles and equipment.

PRACTICAL TIPS

Coping with reflux A baby with reflux will dislike being laid flat on his or her back and needs to be handled carefully after a feeding. The following measures will help reduce regurgitation.

- Change your baby's diaper before the feeding and handle your baby gently and hold him or her upright after the feeding.
- Give smaller feedings more frequently to avoid overloading your baby's stomach.
- If you are bottle-feeding, use a thickened formula, designed for babies with reflux problems. (Ask your doctor for advice.) Don't add extra powdered formula to a feeding. A breast-fed baby over 4 months old can be given 2 teaspoonfuls (10 ml) of baby rice cereal dissolved in 2 tablespoons (30 ml) of expressed milk or formula before feedings.
- Your baby may be more comfortable in a baby seat immediately after a feeding. Raising the head of the crib slightly on books or bricks may help make your baby more comfortable during sleep.

Preventing reflux
Keep your baby semi-upright in a baby chair or seat for the first 30 minutes or so after each feeding.

 ## Seek further medical advice

Arrange to see your doctor if:

- **Your baby appears lethargic or listless or you have concerns about his or her weight**
- **Your baby has symptoms of milk intolerance or allergy, such as diarrhea, vomiting, abdominal pain, and colic**
- **Reflux persists after the age of 18 months**

Sleep problems (babies)

In the first 3 months of a baby's life, night waking is to be expected because all babies need to be fed at night. Some continue to need night feedings for up to 6 months. Sleep problems in these early months tend to center on getting a baby to settle again after a feeding, particularly at night, or the baby waking again after a short time. Older babies who are difficult to put to bed and/or who wake at intervals during the night need a fixed bedtime routine and, sometimes, a period of training in how to fall asleep by themselves and resettle themselves when they wake. Illness, changes in routine, and feeding problems can all affect a baby's sleep temporarily.

 See also **Feeding problems**, pp.144–145; **Colic**, p.148; **Excessive crying**, p.149.

 ## See your doctor first

Arrange to see your doctor if:

- Your baby seems unwell or you are concerned about him or her in any way
- Your baby wakes up suddenly screaming and cannot be consoled

What you can do yourself

Try some or all of the following measures if your baby does not sleep well. Sticking to a routine with your baby and being consistent in your approach will bring results, although it may take time.

Babies up to 4 months

- Keep a sleep journal for a week, noting when and how your baby falls asleep and wakes. This will show whether there is a pattern to sleep disturbance and help you decide on strategies.

- Put your baby to sleep on his or her back, on a firm mattress with no pillow, toward the foot of the crib, so the bedding cannot cover his or her face.

- Check that your baby is not too hot or too cold. Keep the room at about 65°F (18°C) and don't put the crib close to a heater. Don't wrap your baby tightly. Cover him or her with one or two light blankets. Don't use a quilt.

- When your baby wakes for a night feeding, keep the lighting low and change the diaper first or do not change it all unless your baby is very wet or has diaper rash. If your baby falls asleep at the breast or bottle, gently place him or her in the crib. Don't make elaborate attempts to burp the baby or you may wake him or her up again.

 ## PRACTICAL TIPS

Establishing sleep associations

Using the same sequence of events every night will help your baby associate them with falling asleep.

- Bathe your baby at the same time each evening and make this a calm, quiet time, if possible, without too much stimulation and excitement.
- For a baby under 6 months, place the baby on his or her back in an airy crib. Stay beside the crib with your hand resting lightly on his or her chest and sing. Stick to the same song every night since this will now become your baby's sleep association.
- For older babies, sit by the crib spending time with your baby with a book or favorite toy and then settle your baby. Over time, a favorite soft toy, muslin cloth, or blanket may become a transitional object that helps a baby to sleep. Some babies find their own thumb and suck it for comfort.

Transitional object
When a baby begins to associate security and comfort with a favored blanket or soft toy, it becomes a transitional object.

What you can do yourself *continued...*

- You may want to have your baby in bed with you in the early months, especially if you breast-feed, but be aware of the following precautions. You need a wide, firm bed and must lay the baby on the mattress (not on a pillow) with only a light blanket as a cover. Don't sleep with your baby if you or your partner are smokers, have been drinking alcohol, or have taken sleeping pills or other drugs.

- Try to establish good sleep associations early on (*see* PRACTICAL TIPS, opposite page). Carrying and rocking, or a ride in the carriage or car, will help settle a young baby between feedings during the day, but don't use these methods continually or your baby may not be able to sleep without them.

- Encourage longer sleeps at night by establishing the difference between day and night. Keep the curtains open during daytime naps, and play and talk to your baby while you feed and change him or her. Keep the room dark at night and all stimulation to a minimum during and after a feeding.

Babies over 4 months

- Try to establish regular daytime naps because learning to settle and sleep in the day can improve your baby's sleep at night. All babies under a year need two naps of an hour or more each day. Make sure the last nap is early in the afternoon so that it does not interfere with sleep at night.

- If your baby is over 4 months and gaining weight and feeding well, you can teach him or her to sleep better at night. A period of night-time training using controlled crying or gradual withdrawal (*see* PRACTICAL TIPS, right) will stop your baby's sleep problems becoming entrenched. Accept that if you have always comforted your baby promptly when he or she wakes, you are sure to feel anxious about this process at first.

- If your baby over 6 months has partial awakenings in which he or she cries briefly and thrashes around in the crib, check that your baby is well and resettle him or her. Keep a regular routine and prevent overtiredness to avoid the problem.

Seek further medical advice

Arrange to see your doctor if:

- Sleep problems are persisting or any unexplained symptoms develop

PRACTICAL TIPS

Controlled crying You can use this technique to teach an older baby (who no longer needs to be fed during the night) to fall asleep by his or herself at bedtime and to settle again if he or she wakes during the night. You may find the process tough for the first few nights, but try to see it through.

- When your baby cries don't rush in; wait for 5 minutes, then enter the room and say "good night" or "back to sleep now" (choose your own phrase). Then leave, even if your baby is still crying.
- Wait for 10 minutes before you return to your baby and repeat the phrase again in a calm, cheerful tone. Repeat the sequence again after a 15-minute interval, then again after a maximum interval of 20 minutes.
- Now restart the procedure entering the room at 5-, 10-, 15-, and 20-minute intervals. Don't give up if your baby continues to cry. Parents need to support each other through this process since most babies protest vigorously at first.
- Use the same technique consistently each night; it should begin to have an effect within 3–6 days.

Gradual withdrawal If you find controlled crying too difficult, try a separation technique called "gradual withdrawal."

- Place your awake baby in the crib, using your settling routine (*see* PRACTICAL TIPS, opposite page), and sit on a chair near the crib until your baby falls asleep.
- Every 2–3 days, move the chair a little farther from the crib until you are sitting by the door.
- Once you have reached this stage, try settling your baby and leaving him or her to fall asleep alone.

Learning to fall asleep
Your baby may cry vigorously at being left for the first few nights, but if you maintain a consistent approach, he or she will learn to fall asleep alone and to resettle if he or she wakes during the night.

Colic

Colic is used to describe bouts of crying and upset behavior in an otherwise healthy baby. These bouts tend to recur at the same time each day, usually in the early evening, and can last for 3 hours or more. A colicky baby screams and draws up his or her knees, clenches the fists, and appears to have a stomachache. Comforting has little effect. As many as 1 in 5 babies develops colic, usually starting 2–3 weeks after birth, and no one is sure why it occurs. The problem disappears when the baby is about 4 months old and causes no lasting harm, but it is distressing for parents. In a few babies, colic may be due to a cows' milk allergy.

 See also **Feeding problems**, pp.144–145; **Sleep problems**, pp.146–147; **Excessive crying**, opposite page.

 ## See your doctor first

Make an appointment to see your doctor if:

- Your baby's behavior or crying suddenly changes from its normal pattern
- Your baby has a fever, diarrhea, or vomiting
- There is blood in your baby's feces
- Your baby is not gaining enough weight

What you can do yourself

Colic varies from one baby to the next, so try a variety of measures to see which helps.

- If you are bottle-feeding, try changing to a hypoallergenic formula for a week to see if the problem is due to a milk allergy. If you are breast-feeding, exclude dairy products from your diet. If colic improves, continue these measures.

- Too much caffeine in breast milk can make a breast-fed baby irritable, so reduce your intake of coffee and other caffeinated drinks.

- "Pause and burp" your baby at least twice during each feeding, and don't let your baby guzzle. If you are bottle-feeding, check that the hole in the nipple is not too large so the baby gulps, or too small so the baby struggles to feed. You may find an "anticolic" bottle and nipple effective.

 - Experiment with different ways of soothing your baby (*see* PRACTICAL TIPS, right).

- Your baby may pick up on your mood if you are tired and tense. Deep breathing exercises (*see* PRACTICAL TECHNIQUE, p.20) may help you stay calm through a bout of colic.

PRACTICAL TIPS

Calming a colicky baby A colicky baby can be unpredictable so you might need to switch tactics from time to time.

- If your baby is jumpy and oversensitive to stimulation, try a tranquil, orderly bedtime routine, taking time to bathe and feed your baby. Put him or her in a crib in a quiet place, with the lights dimmed.
- Background noise calms some babies, so try putting your baby to sleep with a vacuum cleaner or washing machine running nearby. If your baby can only be calmed by movement, try an outing in the carriage or put him or her in a car seat and go for a drive.
- Enlist help from family and friends during difficult evenings. If you are on your own, put the baby in a sling and sing to him or her while you do other tasks.

Soothing actions
You may find that your baby enjoys being rocked or having you sing to him or her.

 ## Seek further medical advice

Arrange to see your doctor if:

- You find it difficult to cope with the crying
- You think the problem is not due to colic

Excessive crying

Crying is the way a baby communicates its needs, and most young babies cry intermittently for up to 3 hours a day. The usual causes are hunger, discomfort from a wet or dirty diaper, gas, loneliness, being too hot or too cold, or being overtired. As parents learn to recognize types of crying and respond quickly, the baby tends to cry less. However, if you have a baby who cries excessively, he or she will sleep much less than the 16–18 hours that is normal for a newborn baby. Your baby may be difficult to feed, soothe, and settle, and leave you feeling inadequate and exhausted. Most babies grow out of excessive crying by the age of 6 months.

 See also **Feeding problems**, pp.144–145; **Sleep problems**, pp.146–147; **Colic,** opposite page.

 ## See your doctor first

Arrange to see your doctor if:

- Your baby's crying sounds unusual and is accompanied by symptoms such as fever

What you can do yourself

Try the following suggestions to help you cope with a crying baby. Every baby is different, so see what works best for yours.

- If it is more than 2 hours since the last feeding, offer another feeding. Most newborn babies need to be fed every 2–4 hours, day and night. Burp your baby by holding him gently upright on your lap or over your shoulder.

- Change your baby's diaper if it is wet or dirty. You may find your baby becomes calmer if you let him or her kick freely without a diaper for a short time on the changing mat in a warm room.

- Check the back of your baby's neck to make sure he or she is not too hot or too cold. It should be warm and not sweaty, although your baby's hands and feet may be cooler than his or her body. Adjust clothing and covers as necessary.

 - If your baby seems tired but fights sleep, try a settling routine (*see* PRACTICAL TECHNIQUE, right).

- Put a bored or lonely baby in a baby chair so he or she can watch you, or in a sling facing forward.

- When you feel you can't cope, take the baby for a walk or put him or her in a crib, and take a break. Ask a relative or friend to take over for a few hours, and use the time to rest, or do something you enjoy.

 ### PRACTICAL TECHNIQUE

Settling a baby If your baby is happy in your arms and only cries when placed in the crib, you may need to develop a settling technique.

- Try holding your baby in your arms and singing for a few minutes until he or she relaxes. Then gently place your baby in the crib, keeping your hand on your baby's chest and continue singing.
- Stay by your baby for 10 minutes or so until he or she can lie happily in the crib, then move away. If crying resumes, lift the baby, comfort and cuddle him or her, and try again.

Settling technique
Keep your hand on your baby's chest and sing until he or she relaxes and stays calm.

 ## Seek further medical advice

Arrange to see your doctor if:

- **Your baby has developed new symptoms or you are finding it difficult to cope**

Rashes and skin problems

Young babies have sensitive skin that is susceptible to pimples and rashes. Most rashes, such as the tiny white spots (milia) seen on the nose and cheeks of newborn babies, are harmless and clear up quickly. However, a rash may be due to a disorder such as eczema, or an infectious illness, such as chicken pox, measles, or meningitis.

 See also Rubella, p.27; Measles, p.29; Chicken pox, p.32; Eczema, p.38; Heat rash, pp.46–47; Diaper rash, p.152.

WARNING

Seek immediate medical help if your baby has a rash and is:
- Drowsy or floppy and dislikes being touched or held
- Has a fever, a high-pitched cry, and/or is vomiting or refusing food

 ## See your doctor first

Make an appointment to see your doctor if:

- You are unsure what has caused the rash
- Pimples are blistered, crusty, or weepy
- A rash is accompanied by other symptoms

What you can do yourself

The measures below will help you identify and deal with your baby's skin problems.

 • A red or purple blotchy rash should be checked carefully (*see* PRACTICAL TECHNIQUE, right).

• Don't use soaps or wipes on your baby until he or she is at least 6 weeks old, since these can dry the skin; use plain water instead. Add a few drops of baby oil to your baby's bath.

• Wash and dry your baby's face carefully after each feeding to avoid rashes on the chin or cheeks caused by food traces or regurgitated milk.

• Dress your baby with cotton next to the skin; fabrics such as wool can irritate delicate skin.

• Put a muslin cloth over the undersheet in the stroller and crib and change it regularly if your baby dribbles. When holding your baby, use a cloth to stop his or her skin from rubbing against your clothes, and change position occasionally during feedings.

 • If a newborn has dry skin on the hands and feet, rub in moisturizing cream (*see* DRUG REMEDIES, right).

 • If your baby develops a heat rash, cool him or her down (*see* PRACTICAL TECHNIQUE: TREATING A BABY WITH HEAT RASH, p.46).

 ### PRACTICAL TECHNIQUE

Checking a rash A dark red or purple blotchy rash may be a sign of meningitis. Using the glass tumbler test will help you establish whether this is a possibility.

• Press a clear glass firmly against the rash. If the rash does not fade and is still visible through the glass, get medical help immediately.

• If the rash fades, repeat the test again later. In a few cases, a meningitis rash fades at first but later becomes typical and does not fade when pressed.

Possible meningitis
This rash is still visible when the glass is pressed against the skin, so it may be a sign of meningitis.

 ### DRUG REMEDIES

Moisturizers (*see* p.187), such as water-based cream or an unperfumed baby cream, will help moisturize and protect your baby's skin. Apply a cream thinly to the skin after washing your baby.

 ## Seek further medical advice

Arrange to see your doctor if:

- A skin problem does not clear up promptly
- A rash becomes blistered, crusty, or weepy, or your baby develops a fever

Cradle cap

Thick, crusty yellowish scales, known as cradle cap, sometimes develop on a baby's scalp during the first few months of life. The skin may be reddened, and the scales occasionally spread to the baby's forehead and behind the ears. If your baby has hair, you may notice flakes that look similar to dandruff. There is no particular cause for cradle cap, and it is unlikely to bother your baby. However, if he or she has many thick scales, it can look unsightly. Usually, the condition has disappeared completely by the time a baby is 1 year old.

Cradle cap on a baby's scalp

What you can do yourself

Although cradle cap tends to clear up by itself eventually, using these home treatments will help prevent the buildup of scales and improve the appearance of your baby's scalp.

- Wash your baby's scalp every day with a mild baby shampoo, rinse off thoroughly with warm water, then gently dry the scalp with a soft towel.

- After washing your baby's hair, brush the hair and scalp with a soft baby brush to remove the scales. You may find this is enough to clear up a mild case of cradle cap and it will prevent the condition from recurring.

- Massaging your baby's scalp with oil will help to remove thick or crusty scales (*see* PRACTICAL TECHNIQUE, right).

- For more persistent cradle cap, try an anti-dandruff shampoo that contains sulfur and salicylic acid (*see* DRUG REMEDIES, right).

- Don't try to pick off the scales since this may make your baby's head sore.

 ## Seek further medical advice

Arrange to see your doctor if:

- The cradle cap is not getting better after a few weeks of home treatment
- The scales begin to spread to other areas, such as the baby's neck, armpits, or groin
- The rash or the underlying scalp becomes very red or weepy

PRACTICAL TECHNIQUE

Oil treatment Massaging olive oil or baby oil gently into your baby's scalp with your fingers will help loosen cradle cap scales. You can leave the oil on for a few hours or overnight, then shampoo it off afterward. Once your baby's hair has dried, gently brush the hair and scalp with a soft baby brush, and the scales should flake off. Brushing every day may stop the scales from forming again.

Scalp massage
Gently rub the oil into your baby's scalp. This will soften loose scales of skin so they can be brushed away more easily.

DRUG REMEDIES

Sulfur and salicylic acid shampoo (*see* ANTIDANDRUFF SHAMPOOS, p.177) may help to clear cradle cap if your baby has many thick scales of skin on the scalp that are persistent and cannot be removed with oil treatment. Follow the directions on the package carefully. Keep the shampoo out of your baby's eyes.

Diaper rash

Nearly all babies are affected by diaper rash at some time, usually due to urine and feces irritating the skin where it is in direct contact with the soiled diaper. Leaving a baby in a wet or soiled diaper for too long can cause diaper rash, as can a bout of diarrhea. Sometimes the rash is a reaction to new foods in the diet. If your baby has diaper rash, the diaper area will look red and sore, and your baby may be irritable. If the rash becomes infected, it may affect the whole diaper area, including the skin creases around the groin. It will then have a red, glistening appearance with pus-filled pimples and will be extremely sore.

 ## See your doctor first

Make an appointment to see your doctor if:

- The diaper rash looks infected or the skin is broken, cracked, or bleeding
- Your baby has a fever

What you can do yourself

There are several measures you can take to treat diaper rash and prevent infection. Most cases of diaper rash clear up in 3–4 days.

 - Change your baby's diaper often to prevent skin irritation (*see* PRACTICAL TECHNIQUE, right). Newborn babies will need a diaper change at every feeding (at least six a day). While your baby has a rash, change the diaper even more frequently.

- Don't use perfumed skin products or baby wipes, which may contain ingredients that sting sore skin, or soaps, which remove the natural oils from the skin, leaving it more prone to dryness and cracking.

- Wash fabric diapers with a nonallergenic laundry detergent and rinse well.

- If your baby has started solid foods, introduce one new food at a time to see if anything causes a bout of diaper rash.

 ## Seek further medical advice

Arrange to see your doctor if:

- The rash is not clearing up after a week
- The whole diaper area, including the skin creases, becomes affected, or the skin becomes red and hot and pus-filled spots form

 ## PRACTICAL TECHNIQUE

Diaper changing Adopt this diaper changing routine while your baby has diaper rash to help sore skin heal and prevent recurrences.

- When changing the diaper, first wipe away any feces using a dry tissue or cotton balls, and then pour or spray warm water over the area and wipe again. Dab dry with a soft towel.
- Let your baby kick without a diaper on the changing mat for about 10 minutes to expose his or her skin to the air. This helps prevent fungal infections that thrive in dark, damp, warm areas of the body.
- Protect your baby's skin by applying a barrier cream, such as zinc oxide cream (*see* DRUG REMEDIES, below) before putting on a fresh diaper.
- Use a gel disposable diaper that draws away wetness from your baby's skin.

Barrier cream
Apply a thin layer of cream, being careful to protect the skin folds around the top of the legs.

 ## DRUG REMEDIES

Zinc oxide cream (*see* p.189) is often used as a barrier cream to treat and prevent diaper rash. Apply the cream to the diaper area after each wash and diaper change.

FIRST AID

In the following section you will find basic first-aid techniques for minor problems, such as blisters and insect stings, and essential instructions to help you deal with potentially life-threatening injuries and situations, such as choking and shock. Don't wait for an emergency before you refer to these pages because you will be better equipped if you familiarize yourself with the basics now. Although the advice given here may be invaluable in an emergency, it is not intended to be a replacement for the practical training that is given in a first-aid course.

First-aid essentials

To give first aid effectively, it is important to be well prepared. The step-by-step plan given below can be applied to any emergency to help you deal with a victim. Cross-references take you to the specific first-aid techniques you may need on other pages. Access to first-aid materials can make all the difference in an emergency, so an essential kit is described here.

WARNING

If you cannot approach a victim without putting yourself in danger, dial 911 or call emergency medical services (EMS) immediately.

Emergency action plan

The following plan will help you deal calmly, safely, and efficiently with a victim in any situation.

1 Danger Before you act, see if the person is in danger. Deal with any hazards if you can, but do not put yourself in danger to give first aid.

2 Response Find out if the person is conscious (*see* p.168). If he or she is conscious, deal with any injuries. If the person is unconscious, go to the next step of this emergency plan.

3 Airway Make sure that the victim's airway is open and not obstructed so that air can enter the lungs freely (*see* p.168).

4 Breathing Check for breathing. Get someone to dial 911 or call EMS. If the victim is breathing, place him or her in the recovery position (*see* p.169). If not, begin rescue breathing (*see* p.170).

5 Circulation After giving rescue breathing, check for signs of circulation (*see* p.170). If you find no signs of circulation, begin chest compressions (*see* p.171). Deal with any injuries only when breathing and circulation are stable.

Checking a victim
Before you begin to assess injuries, check a victim's response, breathing, and circulation.

FIRST-AID KIT

You can buy a first-aid kit or make up your own and put it in an airtight box or tin. Store the kit in a cool, dry place, out of reach of children, but make sure it is easy to access. Store a washcloth and a blanket with the kit and keep an extra first-aid kit in the car.

Adhesive dressings
These are used to cover small cuts, scrapes, and blisters

Triangular bandage
Used as a sling, this bandage supports an injured limb

Elastic bandages
These apply pressure to a wound or support a sprain or strain

Rolled gauze bandages
These bandages are used for holding a dressing in place

Gauze dressing
This is placed directly on a wound and bandaged in place

Wound dressing
This is sterile and can be used as a dressing or bandage

Tubular bandage and applicator
These are used to dress fingers and toes

Cleansing wipes
Alcohol-free wipes are used to clean wounds when there is no water

Adhesive tapes
Micropore tape or adhesive tape holds dressings in place

Tweezers and scissors
Tweezers are used for splinters; scissors for cutting materials

Disposable gloves
These protect from cross-infection when touching body fluids

Cold pack
This helps reduce swelling in sprains and strains

Blisters

Usually occurring on the feet and hands, blisters are caused by friction or pressure. First the skin becomes red and sore, then fluid collects under the surface in a pale, puffy skin sac. You may get blisters on your heel, sole, or toes from wearing boots or shoes that don't fit well, or that have not been "broken in." Blisters on the hands are often the result of heavy manual work. Most blisters heal quickly: as new skin grows beneath them, the fluid is reabsorbed and the surface dries and peels away.

Seek medical advice

Arrange to see a doctor if:

- You have blisters that were not caused by friction or pressure and/or you have other symptoms
- A blister becomes red, painful, and swollen, and oozes pus or blood
- You have recurrent blisters or blisters that heal very slowly
- You have diabetes

What you can do yourself

Use the following procedure to treat your blister. Protecting it from further rubbing and friction will help it heal.

- Don't burst a blister or cut the skin over it. The skin protects against infection.

- Clean and dry the blister, and protect it with an adhesive dressing (see PRACTICAL TECHNIQUE, right).

- If the blister bursts, don't pick at any loose skin around it. Clean, dry, and dress it, as above, and change the dressing daily until it has healed. Leave the area exposed at night to help it dry out.

PRACTICAL TECHNIQUE

Treating a blister
Treat your blister gently to avoid breaking the skin, and keep it clean and dry to reduce the risk of infection.

1 *Wash the blister carefully with clean water. Gently pat it dry with a clean cotton pad.*

2 *Cover the blister with an adhesive dressing, making sure that the pad is bigger than the blister. Alternatively, use a hydrocolloidal dressing that absorbs fluid from the blister and cushions it. For large blisters, use a sterile dressing secured with adhesive tape.*

PREVENTION

Avoiding blisters The following tips will help protect feet and hands from friction and pressure.

- Wear well-fitting shoes or boots, and break them in slowly. Put padding such as moleskin pads on areas that are likely to rub and develop blisters.
- If you plan to walk long distances, wear close-fitting synthetic inner socks to prevent friction and a second pair of socks on top.
- Use protective gloves for heavy manual work.

Cuts, scrapes, and splinters

Small cuts, scrapes, and splinters are common injuries. Cuts usually bleed for a short time. Scrapes bleed less, but may be painful and have dust and dirt trapped in them. You can often see or feel splinters in your skin or under nails, or you may not notice them until the area becomes red, hot, and painful due to infection. These injuries, though minor, can carry the risk of tetanus, a serious bacterial infection that can be fatal. People are normally immunized against it in childhood but may need boosters as adults. After treating any injury that breaks the skin, check that tetanus immunization is up to date. Seek medical advice if it is more than 10 years since immunization or if you are not sure when the last injection was given.

PRACTICAL TECHNIQUE

Removing a splinter

Most splinters can be removed easily. Your goals are to remove the entire splinter, if possible, and to minimize the risk of infection. Put on disposable gloves first, if available, or wash your hands thoroughly.

1 *Clean the area around the splinter with soap and warm water and pat it dry with a gauze pad. Sterilize a pair of tweezers by passing the ends through the flame of a lighter or match. Allow the tweezers to cool down before you use them.*

2 *Squeeze the skin around the splinter to make the end stick out. Grasp the splinter with the tweezers and gently pull it out, at the same angle at which it entered. Try not to break the splinter.*

3 *Squeeze the skin around the wound to make it bleed a little; this will flush out any remaining dirt. Clean the area again with warm, soapy water, pat it dry, and cover it with an adhesive dressing.*

4 *Seek medical advice if a large splinter cannot be removed easily; the site of the splinter becomes hot, red, swollen, and painful; the victim becomes feverish; and/or the victim is not up to date with tetanus immunization.*

Treating a small wound or scrape

Your main goals when treating a minor cut, scrape, or other wound are to control bleeding and minimize the risk of infection. Before you start, put on disposable gloves, if available, or wash your hands thoroughly.

1 *Control bleeding by pressing a clean gauze pad firmly on the wound. Raise the injured area above the level of the heart, if possible, to reduce the flow of blood to the wound. Most small cuts will stop bleeding within a few minutes.*

2 *Rinse the wound with cool running water. Clear out as much dirt as you can. Use a gauze pad to clean the surrounding skin. Lift out any debris in the wound with the corner of the pad, if necessary.*

3 *Dab the area dry with a clean pad. Cover the wound with an adhesive dressing or adhesive bandage. Do not use cotton balls or any fluffy material that may stick to the wound.*

4 *Seek medical advice if the wound is gaping or deeper than was first suspected; you cannot remove gravel or dirt from the wound; the site becomes hot, red, swollen, and painful; and/or the victim is not up to date with tetanus immunization.*

Severe bleeding

Severe bleeding is likely to be distressing both for the victim and for the person who is assisting. It is usually the result of a serious injury such as a stab wound, a severe blow, or a deep cut. The main priorities are to stop the bleeding then to monitor the victim's condition continually. If a large amount of blood is lost, life-threatening shock may develop.

PRACTICAL TECHNIQUE

Treating severe bleeding

While you wait for medical help to arrive, your immediate priority is to stem the flow of blood. Once you have done this, you need to dress the wound as quickly as possible to reduce the risk of infection. You then need to check that the bandage is not restricting circulation. You should also watch the victim for signs of shock (*see* p.165) and try to prevent or minimize its effects.

1 Call 911. Put on disposable gloves or wash your hands. Apply pressure on the wound with a clean, nonfluffy pad or the palm of your hand. Raise the injury above heart level to reduce blood loss. If an object is embedded in the wound, don't remove it; press firmly on either side of it to push the edges of the wound together.

Keep the injured area raised while you apply pressure

2 Help the victim lie down, keeping the injured part raised above the heart. Continue to apply firm pressure on the wound for up to 10 minutes.

3 Once the bleeding has slowed, cover the wound with a sterile dressing and secure it with a bandage that is tight enough to maintain pressure but not so tight that it impairs the blood supply.

CAUTION: Do not apply a tourniquet. If there is an object in the wound, build up padding on either side, and bandage carefully to avoid pressing on the object.

4 Check the circulation beyond the bandage every 10 minutes. Press on a nail or the skin beyond the bandage until it turns pale, then release the pressure. If the color does not return, or returns slowly, the bandage is too tight. Loosen a tight bandage just a little, making sure the injured part is still supported.

5 If further blood loss occurs, apply a second dressing on top of the first. If blood continues to seep through the top dressing, remove both dressings and apply a fresh one. Bandage firmly, making sure that you are applying pressure accurately over the point of bleeding.

6 Monitor and record breathing, pulse, and level of consciousness regularly. Watch for signs of shock (see p.165) and, if necessary, raise the victim's legs so they are above the level of the heart. If he or she becomes unconscious (see UNCONSCIOUSNESS, p.168), be prepared to begin CPR (see pp.170–171).

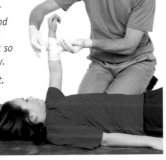

Insect bites and stings

Wasp, hornet, or bee stings are painful, and the site of a sting may be swollen, red, sore, and itchy for a day or two. Flea and mosquito bites develop into itchy red bumps, while a tick (a tiny bloodsucking creature) leaves a swollen, red, beadlike lump on your skin. Ticks can spread disease so they must be removed quickly and carefully. Although most bites and stings are little more than a nuisance, a few people suffer a severe allergic reaction (anaphylactic shock) that needs emergency treatment.

WARNING

Dial 911 or call EMS if:
● There are signs of anaphylactic shock (*see* opposite page)
● You suspect the sting is to the inside of the mouth or throat

What you can do yourself

There are effective techniques for removing stingers and ticks, and remedies that will reduce the general discomfort of bites and stings.

● Watch for symptoms of anaphylactic shock (*see* opposite page). Call 911 if any develop.

● If you suspect a sting to the mouth or throat, call 911. Sucking ice cubes or sipping cold water will help to reduce swelling.

● To treat a sting, remove the stinger, then wash and cool the area (*see* PRACTICAL TECHNIQUE, right).

● If you find a tick, remove it with tweezers. Grasp the head and lever it out, being careful not to leave any of the tick behind. Put the tick in a bottle and see your doctor, taking the tick with you.

● Do not scratch a bite or sting because this will increase the risk of infection.

● Apply an insect bite relief cream or ointment (*see* p.185) to soothe sore, swollen, and/or itchy bites.

● Antihistamine pills (*see* p.178) may help to minimize itching and swelling. You can take medication yourself, but you should not administer it if you are treating someone else.

Seek medical advice

Arrange to see a doctor after 24 hours if:

● Redness and swelling increase
● The bite is oozing or there are red streaks under the skin around the bite

PRACTICAL TECHNIQUE

Treating an insect sting

Follow these steps as soon as possible after the sting has occurred. They will help to reduce immediate pain and swelling and minimize aftereffects such as redness, soreness, and itching.

1 *If you are stung on your wrist, hand, or fingers, remove rings, bracelets, and watches in case swelling develops. If the sting is on a limb, keep it raised to reduce swelling. If you cannot see the stinger, go to step 3.*

2 *Scrape out a stinger that is visible using a firm object, such as a credit card or your fingernail, applying a constant pressure. Don't use tweezers; they may inject more venom into the skin.*

3 *Wash the area with soap and water. Make an ice pack from a bag of frozen peas or crushed ice, wrapped in a towel, or a cloth soaked in cold water and wrung out. Apply it over the site for 10 minutes to reduce pain and swelling.*

Anaphylactic shock

Certain people develop this life-threatening allergic reaction to insect stings, to some foods such as peanuts or shellfish, or to certain drugs. Anaphylactic shock develops within minutes and causes a sudden drop in blood pressure and narrowing of the airways. Symptoms include wheezing; swelling around the eyes and of the face, lips, and tongue; widespread red, blotchy skin eruptions; gasping for air; and anxiety. There is a risk of shock (*see* p.165), and the person may become unconscious.

WARNING

Dial 911 or call EMS.
A person with anaphylactic shock needs urgent medical attention.

PRACTICAL TECHNIQUE

Treating anaphylactic shock

Your goal is to get the victim to a hospital immediately. A person with anaphylactic shock needs emergency medical help, including an injection of epinephrine (adrenaline). People who are susceptible to this type of allergic reaction often carry a prefilled syringe of epinephrine (adrenaline) for self-treatment, but may need your help to use it. While you wait for specialized help to arrive, you should try to ease the victim's breathing, watch him or her carefully for any signs of shock, and treat if necessary.

1 *Call 911. Tell the dispatcher that you suspect anaphylactic shock, and give any information you have on what has triggered the reaction. The victim may be able to give you the details.*

2 *If the victim is conscious, help him or her into a sitting position to make it easier to breathe. Stay calm and be reassuring. Encourage the victim to breathe more slowly and deeply.*

Help the victim to find and use his or her epinephrine (adrenaline) syringe

Sitting up will help the victim to breathe more easily

Support and reassure the victim until help arrives

3 *If the victim has a syringe of epinephrine (adrenaline), help him or her to find and use it, or administer it yourself if you know how to do so.*

4 *Treat for shock (see p.165) if necessary. If the victim loses consciousness but is breathing, put him or her into the recovery position (see p.169). Monitor breathing, pulse, and level of consciousness regularly until help arrives. Be prepared to start CPR (see pp.170–171) if the victim stops breathing.*

Sprains and strains

Sprains and strains are common sports injuries. In a sprain, the ligaments around a joint, such as the ankle, are damaged by overstretching. This is often due to a sudden, unexpected wrenching motion that pulls bones too far apart and tears surrounding tissues. In a strain, the muscles or tendons are overstretched and may be partially torn. The symptoms are much the same for both: there will be pain, swelling, and bruising in the injured limb, and it may feel hot and be difficult to move. Sprains and strains are treated in a similar way and normally improve after a few days, but full recovery may take several weeks.

 ## Seek medical advice

Arrange to see a doctor if:

- You have severe pain, or hear a "pop" at the time of the injury
- You can't put weight on a joint or the injured area looks deformed
- You are concerned about the seriousness of an injury

What you can do yourself

You can treat a minor sprain or strain using the following measures. Start the treatment as soon as possible to reduce symptoms and speed recovery.

 - Follow the **R.I.C.E.** procedure (*see* PRACTICAL TECHNIQUE, right).

- Take acetaminophen (*see* p.177) to relieve pain or ibuprofen (*see* p.185), which also has an anti-inflammatory effect. You can use analgesics to treat yourself, but you should not administer medication if you are treating someone else.

- Keep an elastic bandage or tubular bandage on the limb for the first 48 hours, taking it off at night. Once the bandage is removed, you can start moving the limb gently to the limit of pain-free movement. If there is no reduction in pain and swelling after 2–3 days, seek medical advice.

 ### PRACTICAL TECHNIQUE

R.I.C.E. procedure
The mnemonic **R.I.C.E.** stands for Rest, Ice, Compression, and Elevation, all of which help to speed recovery after a sprain or strain.

1 **Rest** *the injured limb. Avoid any activity that brings on the pain or makes it worse. Sit or lie with the limb in a comfortable position.*

2 **Ice** *reduces pain and swelling. Apply an ice pack (a bag of frozen peas or crushed ice, wrapped in a dry towel or cloth), or a cloth soaked in cold water and wrung out, as soon as possible. Hold for 10 minutes.*

3 **Compression** *involves applying firm, gentle pressure. Put padding on the area and secure it with an elastic bandage. Check that blood flow is not restricted: press a nail or skin beyond the bandage until it turns pale, then let it go. The color should return promptly.*

Apply bandage firmly and evenly

4 **Elevation** *reduces blood flow to the area and minimizes bruising. Raise the injured limb on a stool or cushions. Try not to use the limb for the first few hours after injury.*

Fractures and dislocations

A fracture is a break or crack in a bone due to a heavy blow or a sudden twist or wrench. In open fractures, the bone protrudes through the skin; in closed fractures, the skin is not broken. In a dislocation, the bones of a joint are pulled apart. Signs of a broken bone or dislocated joint include swelling, bruising, and deformity at the site of the injury, and pain and difficulty moving the affected part. A serious fracture, for example of the thigh bone, may cause severe internal bleeding and shock (*see* p.165).

WARNING

Get medical attention immediately if you suspect a broken bone or a dislocated joint. If a person with a broken arm can bend the injured arm, take him or her to the hospital by car. Otherwise, call 911.

PRACTICAL TECHNIQUE

Treating a broken arm
Your main goals are to treat any bleeding, support the injury, and arrange transportation to a hospital. Don't move the person until the arm has been immobilized, unless he or she is in danger. Treat dislocations in the same way. Never attempt to manipulate bones back into place.

1 *If the victim can bend the injured arm, ask him or her to support it. If the bone is protruding from the wound, put on disposable gloves, if available. Cover the wound with a clean dressing. Apply pressure to control bleeding, but don't press on the bone end.*

2 *Make a sling using a triangular bandage, and tie an extra bandage over the sling to keep the arm immobilized against the chest. Don't allow the victim to eat, drink, or smoke in case a general anesthetic is needed in the hospital.*

3 *If the victim cannot bend the injured arm, ask him or her to lie down and put padding around the elbow. Call 911.*

Improvised sling
If no sling is available, turn the edge of the victim's jacket up over the injured arm and attach it to the top of the jacket with a pin.

Treating a broken leg or pelvis
Your main goals are to protect the injured part, call 911, and, for a broken leg, treat any bleeding. Don't move the victim until the injured part has been immobilized, unless he or she is in danger. Never attempt to manipulate the bones back into place.

1 *Call 911. If a bone is protruding, put on disposable gloves, if available, then loosely cover the wound with a clean or sterile dressing. Apply pressure to control bleeding, but be careful not to press on the bone end.*

2 *If the leg is broken, put rolled blankets or coats around the injured leg. Do not let the victim eat, drink, or smoke, in case a general anesthetic is needed in the hospital.*

Put padding around the injured leg

3 *For a broken pelvis, lay the victim down, keeping his or her head low to prevent shock. Place padding around the body, and, if necessary, slip cushions under the knees.*

4 *Monitor and record the victim's breathing, pulse, and level of consciousness regularly. If the pelvis or another large bone is broken, treat for possible shock (see p.165). If he or she becomes unconscious (see p.168), be ready to begin CPR (see pp.170–171).*

Head injuries

All head injuries are potentially serious. A blow to the head may cause a bruise or scalp injury and sometimes a concussion, a brief period of unconsciousness. There is a risk of an underlying skull fracture, as well as compression of the brain from bleeding inside the skull or swelling of injured brain tissues. Symptoms, such as intense headaches, noisy, slow breathing, and drowsiness, may develop hours or even days after the injury. Anyone with a head injury should also be treated for a potential neck (spinal) injury.

> **WARNING**
>
> Call 911 immediately if:
> - There is severe bleeding and/or blood or watery fluid is leaking from the ears or nose
> - A victim loses consciousness

What you can do yourself

You should seek medical advice for all head injuries, even if they are apparently minor.

- For a scalp wound, try to stem any bleeding and dress the injury (*see* PRACTICAL TECHNIQUE, right).

- If there has been a minor blow to the head but there is no bleeding, apply a cold compress (a towel soaked in cold water and wrung out) to reduce swelling and bruising.

- If the victim has a concussion, he or she may feel sick and dizzy and have a headache. Make sure that the victim rests, even if he or she seems to have recovered, and seek medical advice.

- If the victim is conscious but you suspect a more serious head injury, help him or her lie down in a comfortable resting position. Keep the back and neck as still as possible and don't turn the head. Ask simple questions. If he or she seems confused or has difficulty speaking, call 911.

- If the victim becomes unconscious (*see* UNCONSCIOUSNESS, p.168), call 911. Monitor the victim's pulse, breathing, and level of response regularly until medical help arrives or until he or she has recovered.

- If the victim stops breathing, lift the jaw very carefully to open the airway and begin CPR (*see* pp.170–171).

- After a head injury, watch for symptoms such as headaches, weakness, unequal pupil size, and confusion in the hours and days after the injury. Seek immediate medical help if symptoms develop.

PRACTICAL TECHNIQUE

Treating a scalp wound

Bleeding from a scalp wound is often profuse because the area has many small blood vessels. For this reason, a scalp injury may look more serious than it is. If you are in any doubt about the severity of a wound, seek medical advice.

1 *Wear disposable gloves if available, or wash your hands thoroughly. Cover the injury with a clean pad or sterile dressing, pressing firmly on the wound to control the bleeding.*

2 *Bandage the dressing firmly in place. If any blood seeps through it, apply a second dressing on top of the first. If bleeding continues, remove both dressings and apply a fresh one.*

Eye injuries

Eyes are easily bruised or cut by direct blows. They can also be damaged by sharp objects such as fragments of glass, or irritated by grit or dust entering the eye. Chemical splashes may harm the eyes, and many household products, such as detergents, cause irritation if they come into contact with the eyes. An eye injury is usually painful, and the affected eye may water and look swollen and bloodshot. All eye injuries are potentially serious, because there is a risk that vision will be affected.

WARNING

Get emergency medical help if:
- An eye injury causes loss of vision or blurred vision
- An object is embedded in the eye
- A chemical has splashed the eye
- A child has an eye injury

PRACTICAL TECHNIQUE

Treating eye injuries

You should seek medical advice for all but the most minor eye injuries. Your main goals are to keep the victim calm, dress the wound, and get medical help.

1 *Examine the eye carefully. If the victim has a black eye, and you are sure that the injury is not more serious, you may be able to treat it (see BLACK EYE, p.62). A speck of dirt or debris in the eye can be removed as long as it is floating freely on the white of the eye (see FOREIGN OBJECT IN THE EYE, p.61).*

CAUTION: *Don't try to remove debris from the colored part of the eye or remove anything embedded in the eye.*

2 *If the eye has been badly cut or bruised, help the victim lie down and rest his or her head in your lap to keep it still. Tell him or her to try to keep the eyes still. Cover the injured eye with a sterile dressing or clean pad, and ask the victim to hold it in place. Arrange for medical help.*

Treating chemicals in the eye

You must act quickly to wash the chemical out of the victim's eyes. Protect yourself and make sure that the contaminated water drains away freely.

1 *Put on protective gloves, if available. Hold the eye under gently running cold water for at least 10 minutes, positioning the head so that contaminated water does not run into the other eye or down the face. Rinse the eye and eyelid thoroughly. If both eyes are affected, tilt the head to the other side and repeat the procedure.*

Rinse the eye thoroughly

2 *Once the pain has eased, give the victim a sterile dressing or clean pad to hold lightly over the eye. Bandage the dressing loosely in place and take or send the victim to the hospital. Identify the chemical if possible so hospital staff can be informed.*

Burns and scalds

Most minor burns occur in the home – for example, after touching a hot oven or spilling hot water. The skin turns red and the burn feels sore. Deeper burns tend to blister and are usually swollen and painful. Severe burns, which damage deeper layers of skin and sometimes the fat and nerves underneath, may look gray and charred. There may be little or no pain. They cause fluid loss and may lead to shock (*see* opposite page).

 ## Seek medical advice

Arrange to see a doctor if:

- A child has a burn
- A burn is on the hands, face, feet, or genitals
- You are unsure about the severity of a burn
- The burn is an electrical or chemical burn

What you can do yourself

For both minor and more serious burns, it is important to act quickly to make the victim safe and take the heat out of the burn.

Severe burns
- Move the victim away from the source of the heat as quickly as you can.

- Take immediate steps to cool the burn (*see* PRACTICAL TECHNIQUE, right).

- Watch the victim carefully for symptoms of shock (*see* opposite page) and treat if necessary. If the victim becomes unconscious (see p.168), be ready to start CPR (see pp.170–171).

- Take or send the victim to the hospital.

Minor burns

- Take immediate steps to cool the burn (*see* PRACTICAL TECHNIQUE, right).

- While a burn is healing, don't break any blisters that appear. Take acetaminophen (*see* p.177) or ibuprofen (*see* p.185) if the burn is still painful.

- If a burn itches in the later stages of healing, apply moisturizers (*see* p.187) to soothe the skin and prevent it from drying out.

 ### PRACTICAL TECHNIQUE

Cooling a burn
Follow these steps to take the heat out of a burn as soon as possible. Use them for minor burns and to cool a more serious burn while you wait for help.

1 *Hold the burned area under cold running water for at least 10 minutes. If water isn't available, use cold, harmless liquids such as milk or canned drinks. Do not use ice.*

2 *Once the burn has cooled, gently remove anything that might constrict the area if it starts to swell, such as clothing, jewelry, watches, belts, or shoes.*

CAUTION: *Don't try to remove clothing or material that is stuck to burned skin. Cut around the burn and seek medical attention.*

3 *Pat the area dry. Don't put lotions or creams on the burn. Cover it with a sterile, nonadherent dressing or any clean, nonfluffy material, and bandage loosely. Or put plastic wrap lengthwise along the arm to protect the burn.*

Shock

This life-threatening condition occurs when the blood circulation fails, and vital organs such as the brain and heart are deprived of oxygen. The most common cause is severe blood loss, but loss of other body fluids, as occurs in severe burns, can also cause shock. The first signs are a rapid pulse; sweating; and pale, clammy skin. These are followed by a weak pulse; rapid, shallow breathing; thirst; restlessness; and weakness. The victim may become unconscious. If treatment is not given, the heart will stop.

WARNING

Call 911 immediately.
A victim suffering from shock needs urgent medical attention.

PRACTICAL TECHNIQUE

Treating signs of shock

Shock deprives the brain, heart, and other vital organs of oxygen, so the main goals of treatment are to improve the blood supply to the victim's vital organs and to get him or her to the hospital as soon as possible.

CAUTION: Stay with the victim continually, unless you have to leave him or her in order to call 911. Keep the victim still. Do not give anything to eat or drink; if the victim complains of feeling thirsty, moisten his or her lips with a little water.

1 *Call 911. Treat any obvious cause of shock, such as severe bleeding (see p.157) or a burn (see opposite page). Be aware that there may be internal bleeding from an injury such as a major fracture. Gently help the victim to lie down, ideally on a blanket. If his or her legs are uninjured, raise and support them on a chair or on cushions. Keeping the legs higher than the heart and the head low may help to prevent loss of consciousness.*

Use pillows or a pile of folded coats to keep the victim's legs raised higher than the head

Check the victim's pulse regularly until help arrives

2 *Loosen the victim's clothes at the neck, chest, and waist. Cover with a blanket or coat to keep him or her warm, but don't apply a direct source of heat such as a hot-water bottle. Monitor and record his or her breathing, pulse, and level of consciousness regularly. If the victim becomes unconscious, be prepared to start CPR (see pp.170–171).*

Cover the victim completely to keep him or her warm

Seizures

A seizure, also called a convulsion, usually leads to a sudden partial or complete loss of consciousness. During a seizure, the person may cry out and fall, and may go rigid, with an arched back and convulsive movements. The most common cause of seizures is epilepsy, but they may also occur after a head injury, with poisoning (such as from alcohol), or with some brain disorders. In children they are often due to a high temperature; these fits are called febrile seizures (*see* opposite page).

WARNING

Call 911 if:

● A seizure lasts longer than 5 minutes; unconsciousness lasts longer than 10 minutes; multiple seizures occur
● It is a person's first seizure or you suspect head injury or poisoning

PRACTICAL TECHNIQUE

Helping during a seizure

Seizures may look alarming, but most last no longer than a few minutes and do not cause permanent damage. There is little you can do to help the victim to regain consciousness. You can, however, protect him or her from injury; keep a regular check on the breathing, pulse, and level of response during and after the seizure; and arrange emergency help if it is needed.

1 *If you see the victim falling, try to ease the fall by standing behind him or her. Remove any potentially dangerous items, such as hot drinks or sharp instruments, and place them out of reach. Make space around the victim by asking bystanders to move away.*

Place a cushion or soft padding under the head

2 *If possible, protect the victim's head by placing a cushion or soft padding underneath it. Loosen any clothing around the neck. Note the time the seizure started, so you can time how long it lasts.*

CAUTION: *Never try to restrain the victim or put anything in the mouth.*

3 *After the seizure, the victim may fall into a deep sleep. If breathing, put him or her into the recovery position (see p.169). Monitor and record the level of response, pulse, and breathing until he or she recovers. If breathing stops, get someone to call 911 and be prepared to start CPR (see pp.170–171).*

Victim is placed in the recovery position

4 *Call 911 if you are unsure that the victim is prone to epileptic seizures; if he or she is unconscious for more than 10 minutes; convulses for longer than 5 minutes; or has repeated seizures. If none of the above apply, stay with the victim until he or she has recovered completely. Note how long the seizure lasted. Arrange for the victim to get home and suggest that he or she seeks medical advice.*

Febrile seizures

Febrile seizures are fairly common in children, particularly between the ages of 1 and 4 years. In most cases, they are triggered by a high temperature during an illness. At first the child is hot, flushed, and sweaty, the eyes may roll upward, and the child may arch his or her back and clench the fists. He or she may become unconscious, and there may be shaking and twitching of the limbs and body. Normally, the seizure passes quickly, but it is important to cool the child down.

WARNING

Call 911 immediately if a child loses consciousness. Even if the child doesn't become fully unconscious, a doctor must see him or her as soon as possible to rule out an underlying medical condition.

PRACTICAL TECHNIQUE

Helping during a febrile seizure

Although febrile seizures often look alarming, they are unlikely to cause lasting harm to the child if they are dealt with properly and promptly. Your priorities are to protect the child from injury, to cool him or her down, and then to seek medical advice to eliminate any serious underlying causes for the seizure. If the child becomes unconscious at any time during a febrile seizure, call an ambulance.

1 *Place pillows, cushions, or soft padding around the child so that even violent movement will not result in injury. While the child is having a seizure, do not try to move him or her or put anything in the mouth.*

Put rolled-up towels on both sides of the head

2 *Undress the child down to the underpants, and ensure a supply of fresh, cool air by opening a window if possible.*

Gently remove clothing to cool the child

3 *Once the seizure has stopped, encourage the child to lie on his or her side and cover him or her with a light blanket or sheet. When the child wakes, you can give the recommended dose of acetaminophen (see p.177) or ibuprofen (see p.185) if he or she is fully conscious, but only if you are treating your own child. Seek medical advice.*

Put a light cover over the child

4 *If the child loses consciousness briefly (see UNCONSCIOUSNESS, p.168), call 911. Put him or her in the recovery position (see p.169) and monitor and record the level of response, pulse, and breathing regularly until medical help arrives.*

Unconsciousness

Loss of consciousness is potentially life-threatening. It has many possible causes, including a serious injury such as head injury; severe bleeding; shock; poisoning; breathing difficulty; or serious illness. An unconscious victim will not respond to loud noises or to being tapped or shaken, and will not move or make a sound. The eyes may stay closed. If the victim is lying face upward, there is a risk of the tongue blocking the airway, and of choking if he or she vomits. If breathing stops, resuscitation will be needed.

WARNING

Call 911.

A victim who is unconscious needs emergency medical help.

PRACTICAL TECHNIQUE

Helping an unconscious victim

Your priorities are to get emergency medical help and to assess the victim's response, check breathing, and maintain an open airway until help arrives. It is important to prevent him or her from choking on the tongue or on any debris in the airway. You should also look for and treat any obvious injuries and be prepared to resuscitate if breathing stops and/or blood circulation fails.

1 *Speaking loudly and clearly, ask the victim simple questions such as "what is your name?" Tell the victim to open his or her eyes. Gently shake the shoulders (tap the shoulder of a child, or tap the foot of a baby). If there is a response, leave the victim as you found him or her. Call an ambulance, then treat any injuries.*

CAUTION: *Always assume that the victim has a neck injury, and handle him or her very gently.*

2 *If there is no response, shout for help. Open the victim's airway by placing one hand on the forehead and gently tilting the head back. Pick out any obstructions from the mouth and lift the chin with your fingertips. Check whether he or she is breathing, for up to 10 seconds: look for chest movement, listen for breathing sounds, and feel for breath on your cheek.*

Listen for breathing sounds

Watch the chest to detect any movement

3 *If the victim is breathing, place him or her in the recovery position (see opposite page). Look for and treat any obvious injuries, such as fractures (see p.161) or bleeding (see p.157). Monitor and record the level of response, pulse, and breathing regularly until medical help arrives.*

4 *If the victim is not breathing, ask a helper to call 911. Give two effective rescue breaths (see p.170). Check for signs of circulation (breathing, coughing, and movement) for no more than 10 seconds. If they are absent, begin chest compressions (see p.171). When help arrives, describe how the victim was when found and the treatment given.*

PRACTICAL TECHNIQUE

Recovery position (adults and children over 1 year)

If the person is unconscious but still breathing, place him or her in the recovery position, as shown below. This position will keep the body stable, with the head and spine aligned, and will prevent him or her from choking on the tongue or on vomit. It will also keep the airway open and clear. The technique is the same for children over 1 as for adults. (If the victim is found lying on his or her side or front, you can adapt these steps as necessary.)

1 *Kneel beside the victim. Remove any spectacles, and any bulky objects, such as cell phones or keys, from his or her pockets.*

2 *If the victim is on his or her back, place the arm nearer to you at right angles to the body, with the elbow bent and the palm upward. Bring the farther hand across the chest and hold this hand against the cheek. Grasp the thigh farther from you and pull it so that the victim rolls toward you onto his or her side.*

Lay the back of the hand against the face

Grasp the lower thigh, just behind the knee

Let the knee and foot rest on the ground

3 *Once the victim is lying on his or her side, adjust the upper leg so that the hip and knee are bent at right angles. The knee will then support the body. Tilt the head back slightly to keep the airway open, and adjust the hand under the cheek so that the head is supported in this position.*

Recovery position (babies)

● For an unconscious but breathing baby over 1 year, open the airway, then follow the steps described above to place him or her in the recovery position.

● For an unconscious but breathing baby under 1 year, open the airway and cradle him or her in your arms with the head downward. This position will keep the baby's airway open and allow fluids to drain from the mouth.

Hold the baby's head lower than the body

Support the lower body securely

CPR – Rescue breathing

If a victim is unconscious and has stopped breathing, you can supply oxygen to keep him or her alive by blowing your own exhaled air into his or her lungs. This technique, called rescue breathing, is the first stage of cardiopulmonary resuscitation (CPR). Rescue breathing is also used with chest compressions (*see* opposite page) in the second stage of CPR.

WARNING

Call 911.

Send a helper to call 911 if a victim is not breathing.

PRACTICAL TECHNIQUE

Rescue breathing (adults)

Use these procedures to maintain a victim's breathing and circulation until help arrives. If you know a victim has choked, go straight to chest compressions (*see* opposite page).

1 Send a helper to call 911. Make sure the airway remains open by keeping one hand on his or her forehead and two fingers of the other hand under the chin.

2 Pinch the victim's nostrils shut with your thumb and index finger, and open his or her mouth. Take a deep breath, then place your lips around his or her lips, making the most airtight seal you can. Blow steadily into the mouth until you see the chest rise; this usually takes about 2 seconds.

3 Keeping the victim's head tilted, lift your mouth and see if his or her chest falls. If the chest rises and falls, this is an effective breath. If it does not, adjust his or her head. Try again up to 5 times.

4 As soon as you achieve 2 effective breaths, stop and check for signs of circulation (breathing, coughing, and movement) for up to 10 seconds. If signs are present, continue giving 10 breaths per minute until help arrives. Check for circulation every minute.

5 If the victim starts breathing but is still unconscious, place him or her in the recovery position (see p.169). If you can't achieve effective breaths or there are no signs of circulation, go immediately to chest compressions (see opposite page).

Rescue breathing (babies, and children aged 1–7 years)

- Use the adult method for a child aged 1–7 years, but at a rate of 20 breaths per minute instead of 10.
- For a baby under 1, cover the nose and mouth with your lips and give breaths, or breathe into the nose. Give 20 breaths per minute.

CPR – Chest compressions

CPR, or cardiopulmonary resuscitation, is used to resuscitate an unconscious victim who has no signs of circulation, such as coughing, breathing, or movement. If the heart stops beating, blood does not circulate through the body, and vital organs, including the brain, are starved of oxygen. You can maintain some circulation artificially using chest compressions, which help the heart to push blood around the body. Chest compressions are always combined with rescue breathing to ensure that the blood is supplied with oxygen.

PRACTICAL TECHNIQUE

Chest compressions (adults)

The technique combines rescue breaths (*see* opposite page) and chest compressions to simulate circulation.

1 *Call 911. Kneel beside the victim. Place the middle and index fingers of one hand on the notch at the bottom of his or her breastbone.*

Position your hand at the bottom of the breastbone

2 *Place the heel of your other hand on the breastbone next to your fingers. This is the point where you will apply chest compressions.*

3 *Remove the first hand and rest its heel on top of the hand that is in position for chest compressions. Lock the fingers of both hands together firmly.*

4 *Lean over the victim with your arms straight. Press down vertically on the breastbone, depressing the chest by about 1½–2 in (4–5 cm). Release the pressure but don't move your hands. Give 15 compressions at a rate of 100 per minute; then give 2 rescue breaths. Do cycles of 15 compressions and 2 rescue breaths until help arrives or the victim takes a spontaneous breath or makes a movement.*

Chest compressions (babies)

- For a baby under 1 year old, place 2 fingers just below an imaginary line between the nipples and use cycles of 5 chest compressions to 1 rescue breath.

Press down firmly and rhythmically

Chest compressions (children)

- For a child aged 1–7 years, place the heel of one hand on the lower breastbone and use cycles of 5 compressions to 1 rescue breath.

Keep your arm straight during each compression

Choking

When a victim is choking, the airway leading to the lungs is obstructed, often by a piece of food that gets lodged in the airway. Young children and babies are particularly likely to choke on food or something they have put in their mouth. The victim may cough and gasp, get red in the face, have difficulty speaking, and get very distressed. Often, coughing alone is enough to clear the blockage; if it does not, first-aid measures are necessary to prevent loss of consciousness.

WARNING
Call 911 if:
- The person loses consciousness
- You cannot dislodge the blockage successfully using the steps on these pages

PRACTICAL TECHNIQUE

Dealing with choking (adults)
Your main goal is to clear the blockage from the victim's throat as quickly as possible.

CAUTION: Do not put your fingers in the victim's mouth or throat in an attempt to find any trapped object. If you can see an object, pick it out with your finger and thumb.

1 *If the victim is coughing, encourage him or her to keep doing this. If he or she has only a weak cough or stops breathing, stand behind the victim and put both arms around him or her. Make a fist and, with your knuckles facing upward and your thumb toward his or her abdomen, position your fist in the middle of the victim's abdomen, below the ribcage and above the navel.*

Make sure the person is bending well forward

Grasp your fist firmly with your other hand

Put the thumb side of your fist against the abdomen

2 *Grasp your fist with your other hand and pull sharply inward and upward to give abdominal thrusts. Give up to 5 abdominal thrusts, then check the victim's mouth to see if the blockage has been dislodged. Stop thrusts if the airway has been cleared; if not, give 3 further abdominal thrusts.*

3 *If after a further 3 abdominal thrusts, the blockage has not cleared, call 911, and continue to give thrusts until help arrives. If the victim becomes unconscious, get ready to perform CPR (see pp.170–171).*

PRACTICAL TECHNIQUE

Dealing with choking (children aged 1–7 years)

You need to clear the blockage from the throat as quickly as possible. Encourage the child to cough but do not waste time if this is ineffective. You may need to kneel down to use first aid techniques on a child.

1 *Stand or kneel behind the child and bend him or her forward. Place your fist between the navel and the bottom of the breastbone and grasp your fist with your other hand. Pull sharply inward and upward, giving up to 5 thrusts.*

2 *Check the mouth to see if the blockage has been dislodged. Stop thrusts if the airway has been cleared; if not, give 3 more abdominal thrusts.*

Start by placing your fist above the child's navel

3 *If after a further 3 abdominal thrusts, the blockage has not cleared, call 911, and continue to give thrusts until help arrives.*

Grasp your fist with your other hand and pull sharply inward and upward

4 *If the child becomes unconscious while you are waiting for medical help to arrive, get ready to perform CPR (see pp.170–171).*

Dealing with choking (babies under 1 year)

A choking baby may try to cry but instead make strange noises or no sound at all. Use back slaps immediately, then chest thrusts, if necessary.

CAUTION: Never attempt to use abdominal thrusts on a baby under 1 year old.

1 *Lay the baby face down along your forearm, supporting the body and head. Give up to 5 slaps on the baby's back with the palm of your hand. Check the baby's mouth and remove any visible objects with a finger.*

Make sure the baby's head is below level of the chest

2 *If choking persists, lay the baby face upward on your arm. Place 2 fingertips on the lower half of the breastbone just below the level of the nipples. Give up to 5 downward thrusts to the chest. Check the mouth again.*

Push downward on the breastbone with your fingertips

Support the baby's head securely

3 *If chest thrusts fail to dislodge the blockage, repeat the sequence of back slaps and chest thrusts as described above. If the blockage has not cleared after 3 of these sequences, call 911. If the baby becomes unconscious, get ready to perform CPR (see pp.170–171).*

Swallowed poisons

If a poisonous substance is swallowed it can harm the mouth and digestive tract; it may also get into the bloodstream and cause further damage. Household products such as bleach, dishwasher detergent, and paint stripper contain strong chemicals that are poisonous, and many medicines are harmful if taken in excessive doses. Some plants and fungi are poisonous if eaten. The effects of poisoning vary, but there may be vomiting, a burning sensation or pain in the esophagus or abdomen, and loss of consciousness.

WARNING

Call the Poison Control Center 800-222-1222 (US) 800-268-9017 (Can)

A person who has swallowed a poison needs emergency medical attention.

PRACTICAL TECHNIQUE

Dealing with swallowed poisons

The most important step is to arrange medical help. Try to find out what poison was taken, and be ready to resuscitate if the victim becomes unconscious or stops breathing.

CAUTION: Do not try to make the victim vomit, since this could do further harm. If he or she has swallowed a corrosive poison, it will burn the throat again if it is vomited up.

Wipe the mouth carefully to remove traces of poison

1 *Call the Poison Control Center. Try to find out what substance was swallowed and how much has been consumed. Tell the operator; these details will help doctors decide on treatment. If the victim can't tell you what he or she has taken, look for any empty bottles or other items that might suggest what has been consumed; keep them to show the doctor.*

2 *Remove any contaminated clothing and wipe away any remaining poison from around the mouth. Be careful not to get any poison on uncontaminated areas or on your own skin.*

3 *If the lips are burned from a corrosive chemical, give sips of cold milk or water to soothe the mouth and throat. Reassure the victim. If alcohol poisoning is a possibility, cover the victim with a blanket so that he or she doesn't become too cold.*

Encourage the victim to take small, frequent sips of cold milk or water

4 *If the victim becomes unconscious (see p.168), open the mouth and gently remove any substances that you can see. If breathing, put him or her in the recovery position (see p.169). Monitor and record the pulse, breathing, and level of response regularly. Be prepared to perform CPR (see pp.170–171) if necessary.*

A–Z OF DRUG AND NATURAL REMEDIES

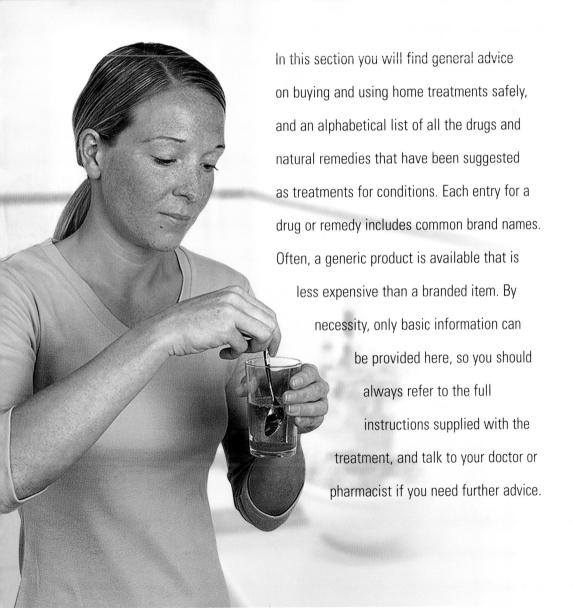

In this section you will find general advice on buying and using home treatments safely, and an alphabetical list of all the drugs and natural remedies that have been suggested as treatments for conditions. Each entry for a drug or remedy includes common brand names. Often, a generic product is available that is less expensive than a branded item. By necessity, only basic information can be provided here, so you should always refer to the full instructions supplied with the treatment, and talk to your doctor or pharmacist if you need further advice.

A–Z of drug and natural remedies

A wide range of medicines is available for home use without a doctor's prescription, as well as many herbal and other natural remedies. Using these safely is an essential part of any home treatment. In this section, you will find information on drugs and natural remedies that have been included in articles in this book, but this is only a basic guide. The advice here is not intended to replace the guidance of medical professionals, so always consult a doctor or pharmacist if you need more information. It is also essential that you read and follow the instructions provided with any drug or remedy and pay particular attention to cautions.

How to use this section

Drugs and natural remedies are listed here alphabetically, and there are cross-references to them from the articles in which they are mentioned. Natural remedies are indicated by a leaf symbol and drug entries by a pill symbol.

At the beginning of each drug entry there is a list of selected common brands with the main ingredients of each brand given in brackets. Where a drug has several applications, the brands for different uses are shown.

Some basic instructions on method of use are provided, but details may vary from one product to another, so always refer to information supplied with the product. Common side effects, if any, are given. Under precautions, you will find concerns that apply when using the product, specific circumstances in which it should not be used, and a cross reference to the GENERAL CAUTIONS (below) when applicable.

General cautions

Although many of the medicines included here can be used safely by most people most of the time, there are situations when extra care is needed or when some treatments should be avoided entirely. Listed below are general cautions that apply when taking medicines and natural remedies. You should also read and follow the instructions and cautions included with the product.

● If you are pregnant or breast-feeding, consult a doctor or pharmacist before using any drug or remedy.

● Speak to your doctor or pharmacist before using a medicine if you have liver or kidney problems or any other chronic medical condition, such as a stomach ulcer, diabetes, heart disease, or high blood pressure. Drugs and remedies may have stronger or different effects because of a chronic illness.

● Before treating babies and children, make sure you are certain of the diagnosis and the suitability of the medicine. Check dosages for different age ranges. Consult your doctor or pharmacist first if you are in doubt about the treatment.

● If you are already taking prescribed medication, talk to your doctor before taking a new drug or remedy. Over-the-counter drugs and natural remedies can interact with each other and with prescribed medicines, sometimes with potentially harmful results. However, don't stop taking prescribed medicine without first consulting your doctor.

● Store medicines and remedies in a cool, dry place, out of reach of children. Check expiration dates and dispose of any medicines and remedies that are out of date.

Using natural remedies safely

Although there is a huge variety of natural remedies available in pharmacies and health stores, only a small number appear in this book. Those that have been included have been selected on the basis that they have undergone medical testing and there is some evidence of their safety and effectiveness. The few exceptions are herbal teas and sleep remedies that may help and are unlikely to cause harm.

A concern when using natural remedies is that much of the evidence for them is anecdotal, and testing of them is usually less rigorous than for conventional drugs. In addition, quality and dosages are not regulated or standardized, so there is no guarantee of their strength, purity, and safety, and their effects cannot be predicted exactly. When buying natural remedies, always use a reputable supplier and make sure there are full instructions and warnings with the product. Observe these carefully and don't exceed the recommended dose.

When taking any remedy, be aware that although many of them are derived from plants and have the label "natural" or "herbal," they are not natural to the human body and can have effects that are as strong as those of conventional drugs. Natural remedies can also interact with other drugs and substances, such as alcohol. Cautions also apply in the same circumstances as conventional drugs (see GENERAL CAUTIONS, left).

Acetaminophen

Common brands

FOR ADULTS ● Tylenol ● Aspirin-Free Anacin ● Bayer Select Maximum Strength Headache Pain Formula
FOR CHILDREN ● Infants' Tylenol Concentrated Drops (2–3 years) ● Children's Tylenol Suspension Liquid (2–11 years) ● Junior Strength Tylenol Chewable Tablets (6–12 years)

Widely used analgesic for toothache, headache, earache, muscle pains, and to reduce fever. Suitable for people with stomach problems since less irritating than aspirin; also during breast-feeding because traces in breast milk are too small to harm a baby.

Method of use Available as regular, soluble, or chewable tablets; or liquid medicine. When treating a child, be careful to choose the correct product for the child's age (*see* COMMON BRANDS, above).

Side effects Usually none.

Precautions Don't give to babies under 2 years, except on a doctor's advice.

WARNING

Don't take with other drugs containing analgesics, such as cold remedies, due to risk of overdose. In case of possible overdose, seek immediate medical attention, even if you feel no ill effects. There is risk of delayed, serious liver damage. Do not drink alcohol while taking acetaminophen.

Aloe vera

The aloe plant (*Aloe vera*) is a centuries-old remedy for skin conditions such as sunburn and psoriasis. May help relieve pain and swelling and speed healing.

Method of use Available in skin creams, gels, and ointments. Apply as needed.

Side effects Usually none.

Precautions None.

Aluminum chloride

Common brand
● Certain Dri

Controls excessive sweating by blocking sweat ducts; use when other methods do not help.

Method of use Available as roll-on applicator. Apply sparingly to clean, dry skin before going to bed. It will not wash off the next day, even if you bathe or shower. One application may prevent sweating for up to 3 days, or longer.

Side effects Possible skin irritation. Stop using if this occurs.

Precautions Don't use on irritated or broken skin, or near the eyes. Don't use after shaving or using depilatories.

Antacids

Common brands

MIXTURES OF CHEMICAL COMPOUNDS: ● Maalox Quick Dissolve Chewable (calcium carbonate) ● Mylanta Antacid Gelcaps (calcium carbonate, magnesium hydroxide) ● Rolaids Antacid Tablets (calcium carbonate, magnesium hydroxide)
WITH SIMETHICONE: ● Gas-X Extra Strength (calcium carbonate, simethicone) ● Maalox Liquid Antacid/Antigas (aluminum hydroxide, magnesium hydroxide, simethicone) ● Mylanta Antacid Anti-Gas Liquid (aluminum hydroxide, magnesium hydroxide, simethicone) ● Riopan Plus (magaldrate, simethicone)

Relieve indigestion or heartburn by neutralizing stomach acid. Contain compounds such as aluminum hydroxide, calcium carbonate, or magnesium hydroxide, or combinations of these. Some also contain simethicone to absorb excess stomach gas.

Method of use Available as hard or chewy tablets, carbonated drinks, or soothing liquids. Method of use varies; follow instructions on package.

Side effects Usually none.

Precautions Antacids can interfere with absorption of some drugs; check with a doctor or pharmacist before use if already taking other medicines. *See also* GENERAL CAUTIONS, opposite page.

Antidandruff shampoos

Common brands
● Neutrogena T/Gel (coal tar) ● Nizoral Shampoo (ketoconazole) ● Polytar AF (coal tar, pyrithione zinc) ● Selsun Blue (selenium sulfide) ● Sebulex (sulfur, salicylic acid)

Selenium sulfide and pyrithione zinc shampoos reduce overgrowth of a type of fungus living on the scalp, a common cause of dandruff. Ketoconazole, an antifungal drug, is very effective, often when other treatments don't work. Coal tar shampoos (*see* p.180 reduce scaling, as does sulfur and salicylic acid which may also be used to treat cradle cap in babies.

Method of use As directed. Beneficial effect may not be apparent for a few weeks.

Side effects Occasionally, itching, irritation, or burning sensation on the scalp.

Precautions Avoid eyes and inflamed or broken skin. Coal tar shampoos may stain blonde or gray hair; may also increase the risk of sunburn for up to 24 hours; protect your head from strong sunshine. *See also* GENERAL CAUTIONS, opposite page.

Antidiarrheal drugs

Common brands
● Pepto Diarrhea Control (loperamide) ● Imodium (loperamide)

Diarrhea is best left to run its course, but when essential, medicines may be taken as a short-term measure to slow bowel activity.

Method of use Use as needed. Take the lowest dose that helps. Drink plenty of clear fluids to prevent dehydration.

Side effects Usually none; loperamide, however, may cause constipation, nausea, fatigue, dry mouth, or a rash.

Precautions *See* GENERAL CAUTIONS, p.176.

Antifungal drugs

Common brands
RINGWORM AND ATHLETE'S FOOT: ● Lamisil Cream (terbinafine hydrochloride) ● Micatin (miconazole) ● Lotrimin (clotrimazole)
VAGINAL YEAST: ● Gyne-lotrimin (clotrimazole) ● Monistat (miconazole nitrate)

Treat fungal conditions, such as ringworm, athlete's foot, or vaginal yeast.

Method of use Cream, powder, or spray powder for skin infections. As suppositories or cream (with applicator) for vaginal yeast. Wash hands after use.

Side effects Occasionally, irritation and redness may occur; if severe, stop using and consult a doctor.

Precautions Avoid eyes, nose, mouth, or broken or sensitive skin. Vaginal suppositories and creams may damage latex condoms and diaphragms. *See also* GENERAL CAUTIONS, p.176.

Antihistamine/decongestant eye drops

Common brands
● Aller-chlor (chlorpheniramine) ● Naphcon A (pheniramine, naphazalone) ● Visine A (pheniramine, naphazalone)

Contain an antihistamine, pheniramine, and a decongestant, naphazalone. Act quickly to provide temporary relief of itchy, red, and watery eyes associated with hay fever and other causes of allergic conjunctivitis.

Method of use Use as directed; usually 1 to 2 drops in the affected eye(s) up to 4 times a day.

Side effects Some users may experience a brief tingling sensation in the eye.

Precautions Remove contact lenses before use. Consult your doctor first if you have urinary problems or glaucoma.

Antihistamines

Common brands
NONSEDATING: ● Allegra (fexofenadine) ● Claritin (cetirizine)
SEDATING: ● Benadryl (diphenhydramine) ● Phenergan (promethazine) ● Phenergan Nighttime (promethazine)

Control allergic symptoms such as sneezing and runny nose. Also itchy eyes, and itchy and inflamed skin from insect bites or nettle rash. Sedative types can be used as a short-term sleeping aid.

Method of use Pills and liquids taken as soon as allergic reaction occurs, or to prevent one. Some need to be taken several times a day; newer types usually only once a day.

Side effects Older, sedating types may cause drowsiness for a few days. Newer nonsedating types less so, but caution needed.

Precautions Don't take sedating types if driving or operating hazardous machinery. *See also* GENERAL CAUTIONS, p.176.

Antinail-biting lotions

Common brands
- Orly No Bite • Super Nail Bite No More

Help stop nail biting. Contain bitter-tasting, but harmless, chemicals.

Method of use Apply directly to nail surfaces. Use every day.

Side effects Usually none.

Precautions Don't use on broken or sensitive skin, and avoid eyes and lips. Check instructions before use on children.

Aspirin (acetylsalicylic acid)

Common brands:
- Bayer • Bufferin • Anacin

Relieves mild to moderate pain in conditions such as migraines, sore throat, toothache, and joint pain and inflammation. Reduces fever. Included in medicines for colds, flu, menstrual cramps, and joint and muscle aches.

Method of use Coated or regular pills, or chewable pills. Take with or after food.

Side effects Indigestion due to irritation of the stomach lining; less likely with coated pills.

Precautions Consult a doctor first if you have or have had asthma or a stomach disorder. Don't use if you are allergic to aspirin or other anti-inflammatory drugs. *See also* GENERAL CAUTIONS, p.176.

WARNING
Before children and teenagers use this medication for chicken pox or flu syndromes, a doctor should be consulted about Reye's syndrome, a rare but serious illness reported to be associated with aspirin.

Baking soda

Baking soda is sodium bicarbonate. It is commonly used in cooking. Can soothe itching and soreness.

Method of use Add 4 tablespoons (or a teacup) to a bath two-thirds full of lukewarm water and soak for about 20 minutes. For soreness inside the mouth, add half a teaspoon of sodium bicarbonate to 1 cup (250 ml) of warm water to make a mouthwash.

Side effects Usually none.

Precautions None.

Benzoyl peroxide

Common brands
- Clearasil Maximum Strength Medicated • Benoxyl 5 Lotion • Neutrogena Acne Mask 5

Preparations for mild or moderate acne reduce inflammation and bacteria and make skin less oily.

Method of use Available as gels, lotions, or creams. Wash skin first. Start with low strength; move on to a higher strength only if needed.

Side effects Skin may redden, peel, and become dry and irritated, but this normally resolves in a few days if treatment is stopped temporarily; if not, use less frequently; if severe, stop using.

Precautions Don't apply to damaged skin. Avoid eyes, lips, mouth, and lining of nose. Benzoyl peroxide can bleach hair and clothes.

Calamine lotion

Common brands
- Calamine Lotion • Calamox

Has a cooling effect and is used to soothe minor skin irritation and rashes.

Method of use Available as lotion or cream. Apply as often as needed. Dab lotion on to skin with cotton balls and let dry.

Side effects Usually none.

Precautions Usually none.

Calendula cream

Creams prepared from extracts of pot marigold, or calendula (*Calendula officinalis*), traditionally used to soothe cuts, scrapes, and mild skin inflammation.

Method of use Available in creams or lotions. Apply as directed on packet.

Side effects *See* GENERAL CAUTIONS, p.176.

Precautions Usually none.

Coal tar preparations

Common brands

CREAMS AND LOTIONS: ● Tegrin Lotion for Psoriasis ● Doak Tar Lotion

SHAMPOOS: ● Tegrin Medicated Cream Shampoo ● T-Gel Therapeutic Shampoo

BATH ADDITIVES: ● Balnetar Therapeutic Tar Bath ● Cutar Water Dispersible Emollientar ● T/Derm Tar Emollient

Used in conditions such as psoriasis to reduce inflammation and scaling. Available as a cream, lotion, shampoo (*see also* ANTIDANDRUFF SHAMPOOS, p.177), or bath additive.

Method of use Apply cream or lotion to clean skin. Wash hands after use. Add products to a warm bath. Pat skin dry. Use shampoos as directed.

Side effects Coal tar can irritate skin or cause a rash. If this occurs, stop using.

Precautions Don't use on broken skin or inflamed or infected psoriasis. Avoid eyes and lining of nose and mouth. Avoid exposing skin to sunlight.

Cold and flu remedies

Common brands

● Actifed Cold and Sinus Caplets (acetaminophen, pseudoephedrine, chlorpheniramine maleate, dextromethorphan) ● Alka-Seltzer Plus Cold and Cough Liqui-Gels (acetaminophen, pseudoephedrine, chlorpheniramine maleate, dextromethorphan) ● Tylenol Flu Maximum Day Strength (acetaminophen, dextromethorphan, pseudoephedrine) ● Sudafed Multi-Symptom Cold & Cough (acetaminophen, dextromethorphan, guaifensin, pseudoephedrine)

Help relieve headache, fever, sore throat, cough, and blocked nose or sinuses. May contain an analgesic, such as acetaminophen (*see* p.177), which also helps reduce fever; a decongestant, such as pseudoephedrine (*see* p.181), to help unblock nose and sinuses; an antihistamine, such as chlorpheniramine (*see* opposite page), for a runny nose; cough suppressants, such as dextromethorphan (*see* p.180); and expectorants, such as guaifenesin.

Method of use Available as pills, liquid, or soluble powders.

Side effects See entries for ingredients.

Precautions *See* GENERAL CAUTIONS, p.176.

WARNING

Don't take remedies containing analgesics with other analgesics due to risk of overdose. Don't take remedies containing decongestants if you have taken MAOI antidepressants in the last 14 days.

Corn and blister bandages

Common brands

● Dr. Scholl's Cushlin Gel Corn Wraps Non-Medicated ● Band-Aid Advanced Healing Blister Cushions ● Curad Advanced Blister Care Gel Bandages

Dressings for blisters contain a substance that absorbs moisture to form a gel that cushions and protects. Types for corns and calluses also soften hard skin to aid removal. Blister dressings keep skin moist (helping it heal), and relieve pain and pressure.

Method of use Choose bandage that covers whole area. Leave on until it comes off itself.

Side effects Usually none.

Precautions None.

Cough suppressants

Common brands

● Robitussin DM (guaifenesin USP, dextromethorphan) ● Benylin Adult Formula Cough Suppressant (dextromethorphan) ● Triaminic Cough (dextromethorphan, pseudoephedrine)

Dextromethorphan remedies for a dry, irritating cough, not for coughs that produce mucus. Suppressants may also contain decongestants, such as pseudoephedrine (*see* right).

Method of use Usually liquids. Take as directed; for coughing at night, take at bedtime.

Side effects Dextromethorphan may cause dizziness, nausea, or stomach upsets.

Precautions Don't take with alcohol. If drowsy, don't drive or use hazardous machinery. Consult doctor before use if you have glaucoma, or prostate, kidney, or liver problems. *See also* GENERAL CAUTIONS, p.176.

WARNING

Don't take remedies containing decongestants if you have taken MAOI antidepressants in the last 14 days.

Counterirritants

Common brands
● Icy Hot (methyl salicylate, menthol) ● Deep Heating (methyl salicylate, menthol) ● Flexa 11454 (menthol) ● Heet (methyl salicylate, camphor, oleoresin capsicum) ● Absorbine Jr. Pain Relieving Liquid (menthol)

Produce a mild tingling in the skin to soothe pain and stiffness in muscles and joints temporarily. Some products warm and increase blood flow to the area; others have a cooling effect.

Method of use Massage cream or apply spray to the affected area. Wash hands after use.

Side effects Occasionally, irritated or reddened skin; if affected, stop using.

Precautions Avoid eyes and sensitive or broken skin. *See also* GENERAL CAUTIONS, p.176.

Cromolyn sodium

Common brands
● Nasalcrom Nasal Spray

Used to help prevent or relieve symptoms of hay fever and other allergic causes of runny nose. Works by preventing release of histamine from the nasal lining which is responsible for causing symptoms of sneezing, itching and runny nose.

Method of use For best results, start using a week or two before the start of the hay fever season and use continuously throughout the season.

Side effects May briefly irritate lining of your nose and also cause sneezing, but this generally settles after a day or two of use.

Precautions Do not use to treat a cold or sinus symptoms.

Cystitis pain relief preparations

Common brands
● Uristat (phenazopyridine)
● Azo Standard (phenazopyridine)

Helps relieve the pain and burning sensation associated with cystitis. Also helps relieve the urgent need to urinate. Phenazopyridine will not cure cystitis and provides only temporary relief. You may still need to see your doctor for treatment.

Method of use Follow directions carefully. Usually, take 2 tablets 3 times a day, after meals as needed. Don't take more than 12 tablets in 2 days.

Side effects Possible headache, dizziness, stomach upset. Urine may turn red-orange or brown; this is harmless.

Precautions Phenazopyridine is for temporary relief of cystitis symptoms. It is not an antibiotic and will not cure the infection.

Decongestants

Common brands
● Non-Drowsy Sudafed Nasal Decongestant Tablets (pseudoephedrine) ● Afrin Nasal Spray (oxymetazoline) ● Vicks Sinex 12-hour Nasal Spray (oxymetazoline) ● Vicks Sinex Nasal Spray (phenylephrine) ● Tylenol Allergy Sinus Medication (chlorpheniramine, pyrilamine, acetaminophen) ● Actifed Cold and Sinus (chlorpheniramine, pyrilamine, acetaminophen)

Fast-acting medications to help relieve nasal and sinus congestion due to of colds, sinusitis, and hay fever for up to 12 hours.

Method of use Apply drops or spray directly into each nostril; with spray, sniff as vapor is released. Take pills and liquid medicine orally.

Side effects Occasionally, stinging, itching, or sneezing may occur.

Precautions Don't use sprays or drops continuously for more than 7 days. Consult a doctor if you are taking prescribed drugs or have diabetes, heart disease, or high blood pressure.

WARNING
Don't take decongestants if you have taken MAOI antidepressants in the last 14 days. *See also* GENERAL CAUTIONS, p.176.

Earwax drops

Common brands
● Murine Ear Wax Removal System Ear Drops (carbamide peroxide) ● ERO Ear Wax Removal Drops (carbamide peroxide) ● Bausch & Lomb Ear Wax Removal System (carbamide peroxide)

Used to soften, loosen, and remove excess earwax.

Method of use Tilt head and apply drops into ear. Treat one ear at a time, a few days apart.

Side effects May cause brief "bubbling," mild stinging, and irritation in the ear.

Precautions Don't use if there is pain, inflammation, or damage in the ear, a burst eardrum, dizziness, or recurrent ear problems. For occasional use only.

Echinacea

Herbal remedy believed to help the body fight infections. Used at the start of a cold, may help to reduce symptoms and speed recovery.

Method of use Available as capsules, tea, fresh-pressed juice, or a tincture.

Side effects Uncommon; the most likely problems are stomach upset and nausea.

Precautions Don't use for more than 8 weeks; may worsen asthma or cause allergic reactions. *See also* GENERAL CAUTIONS, p.176.

Essential fatty acids

Essential fatty acids (EFAs), particularly omega-3 EFAs, help the body to form healthy cells and nerve tissue; may also help relieve depression and affect hormones that contribute to menstrual cramps and PMS.

Method of use Found in foods, principally oily fish such as sardines and salmon; olive oil; walnuts; and flax seeds.

Side effects Usually none if EFAs are eaten as part of a balanced diet.

Precautions None.

Essential oils

Eucalyptus, camphor, and menthol used externally for treating colds and blocked sinuses. Inhaling vapors helps unblock the nose and ease breathing.

Method of use Oils, chest rubs, and lozenges. Inhale a few drops of oil placed on a tissue; at bedtime, place tissue inside the pillowcase. Apply a rub to the chest, throat, and back. Suck menthol lozenges to relieve a stuffed-up nose.

Side effects Usually none.

Precautions Never ingest essential oils. Some may not be suitable for children or for use during preganancy.

Eye lubricants

Common brands
EYE DROPS: ● Artificial Tears (hydroxypropyl methylcellulose) ● Tears Naturale (hydroxypropyl methylcellulose) ● Lubricating and rewetting eye drops for contact lens wearers (sodium chloride) GELS: ● GenTeal (hydroxypropyl methylcellulose) OINTMENT: ● Lacri-lube (mineral oil, white petrolatum)

Drops and gels keep eyes moist and relieve itching and dryness. Ointment containing white petrolatum lubricates eyes at night.

Method of use Always wash hands before use. Apply inside lower eyelid. Keep droppers or nozzles away from eyeball or any other surfaces.

Side effects Brief stinging or blurred vision.

Precautions If vision is blurred, don't drive or use hazardous machinery. Some eyedrops contain chemicals that can damage contact lenses; never wear contact lenses when using ointment. Try to avoid using ointment in daytime since it may blur vision.

Feverfew

Feverfew (*Tanacetum parthenium*) is a garden herb found by some people to reduce the frequency and severity of migraine attacks.

Method of use Available as capsules, pills, leaf powder, or tea.

Side effects Usually none; most likely problems are mouth inflammation or ulcers. If taken for long periods and stopped suddenly, "rebound" headaches, anxiety, disturbed sleep, and palpitations may occur.

Precautions Don't take if you are pregnant (may cause miscarriage) or breast-feeding. *See also* GENERAL CAUTIONS, p.176.

Flatulence relief

Common brands
● Gas-X (calcium carbonate, simethicone) ● Maalox Max (calcium carbonate, simethicone) ● Maalox Anti-Gas (simethicone) ● Flatulex (activated charcoal, simethicone)

Simethicone breaks down bubbles of gas in stomach. Sometimes combined with an antacid (*see* p.177) or with charcoal in preparations to treat indigestion.

Method of use As directed on package. Available as hard pills, chewable pills, and liquid.

Side effects Usually none.

Precautions Consult your doctor before giving flatulence relief preparations to a child.

Ginger

Common spice and flavoring. Ginger (*Zingiber officinale*) may also help to prevent or relieve nausea in conditions such as motion sickness.

Method of use Available as capsules, candies, or tea. Can be eaten fresh, crystallized, or powdered in capsules or tea. To help prevent motion sickness, take 30 minutes before journey.

Side effects Brief heartburn or gas.

Precautions None.

Ginkgo

May improve circulation: in particular, blood flow in the brain to help relieve tinnitus.

Method of use Available as pills, tincture, or capsules. Beneficial effects may take 4–6 weeks.

Side effects Mild stomach upset or nausea may occur.

Precautions May increase risk of bleeding. Don't take with blood-thinning drugs, or if you are pregnant. *See also* GENERAL CAUTIONS, p.176.

Glucosamine and chondroitin

Naturally occurring substances in cartilage covering bone ends in joints. In arthritis, supplements of either or both may help relieve pain, improve flexibility, and slow rate of damage.

Method of use Usually taken as pills. Full effects may take at least a month; if there is no improvement after 10 weeks, stop using.

Side effects Usually none.

Precautions Don't take glucosamine if you are allergic to shellfish. Consult a doctor before use with blood-thinning drugs such as warfarin, or if you have diabetes. *See also* GENERAL CAUTIONS, p.176.

H2-blockers

Common brands
● Tagamet (cimetidine) ● Zantac 75 (ranitidine)

Reduce amounts of stomach acid to relieve occasional bouts of indigestion and heartburn. Especially useful if antacids (*see* p.177) have not helped.

Method of use Follow instructions carefully. Recommended only for short-term use (no more than 2 weeks).

Side effects Usually none; most likely problems are headaches, dizziness, stomach upsets, rash, and fatigue.

Precautions Not usually recommended for children under 16. *See also* GENERAL CAUTIONS, p.176.

Hair bleaches

Common brand
● Jolen Creme Bleach (hydrogen peroxide)

Mild bleach used to lighten facial or body hair and make it less noticeable against fair skin.

Method of use Usually a cream supplied with ammonia to activate bleach. Mix and apply with a spatula. Use as directed on the packet.

Side effects Irritation or allergic reaction may occur; test on a small area of skin. Wait for 24 hours to make sure there is no reaction.

Precautions Don't use on broken or inflamed skin or near the eyes. Don't use after taking a bath, since skin is sensitive, or expose treated areas to sunlight for 24 hours. Can stain clothing and furniture.

Hair-removal products

Common brands
● Nair Roll-on ● Neet ● Nair Microwave Wax Kit

Creams and mousses dissolve hair down to the roots. Wax and "sugaring" preparations pull out hairs, so effect lasts a couple of weeks.

Method of use Creams applied with a spatula. Mousses sprayed on and then washed off. Waxes and sugars applied to clean, dry skin with hairs at least ¼ in (5 mm) long; fabric strips applied and pulled off against direction of hair growth.

Side effects Creams and mousses may cause irritation; if so, wash off immediately. Waxes and sugars may produce raised, red spots briefly.

Precautions Can cause allergic reactions; test on small area first. Don't use on irritated or broken skin, on moles or warts, or within 2 hours of bathing or sunbathing. Wait 24 hours before using deodorants or perfumes. Avoid waxes or sugars if you have diabetes.

Head lice preparations

Common brands
● Acticin (permethrin) ● Nix Cream Rinse (permethrin)

Antiparasitic treatments for head lice infestations.

Method of use Available as shampoos or lotions. Lotions are more effective than shampoos.

Side effects Can irritate skin, causing redness and stinging.

Precautions Avoid broken or infected skin, and eyes. Check suitability before using on small children or babies.

Hemorrhoid preparations

Common brands:
● Preparation H (glycerin, petrolatum, phenylephrine, shark liver oil) ● Tucks Hemorrhoid Pads with Witch Hazel ● Anusol HC-1 (hydrocortisone acetate)

Some preparations contain hydrocortisone to relieve anal itching and inflammation, or phenylephrine to shrink swollen tissue. Witch hazel wipes are cooling and soothing. Cream preparations lubricate the area, making it easier to pass stools.

Method of use Available as cream, ointment, suppositories, or pads. Clean and dry anal area before use. Wash hands before and afterward.

Side effects May sting as they are applied.

Precautions Don't use for more than 5–6 days, as may irritate anal skin; if hemorrhoids persist, see a doctor. Some brands unsuitable for children. Witch hazel pads are for external use only.

Herbal sleeping remedies

Herbs such as valerian (*Valeriana officinalis*), hops (*Humulus lupulus*), passionflower (*Passiflora incarnata*), and chamomile (*Matricaria recutita*) are said to aid relaxation and sleep.

Method of use Available as pills or liquid, taken at bedtime. Chamomile can be drunk as tea. Pillows stuffed with dried hops are also available. Try pills and liquids for only a few days at a time. If sleeping problem persists, consult a doctor.

Side effects Usually none.

Precautions None.

Herbal teas

Chamomile or fennel seed teas traditionally used to relieve indigestion, heartburn, or gas; ginger tea (*see* p.183) used for nausea and motion sickness; chamomile tea for insomnia (*see* HERBAL SLEEPING AIDS, above).

Method of use Add boiling water to a teaspoon of herb, and brew for a few minutes. Don't add milk.

Side effects Usually none.

Precautions None.

Hydrocortisone cream

Common brands
● Cortaid ● Lanacort

Mild steroid cream reduces inflammation in non-infectious conditions, such as eczema, insect stings, and skin reactions to jewelry, plants, and toiletries. Also in some hemorrhoid preparations (*see* p.182).

Method of use Apply thinly as directed on packet. Don't put dressings over treated area.

Side effects Usually none.

Precautions Don't use for longer than a week. Don't use on the face, genital area, or broken or infected skin. Don't use on children under 2 years, unless on doctor's advice. *See also* GENERAL CAUTIONS, p.176.

Ibuprofen

Common brands
FOR ADULTS: ● Advil ● Motrin
FOR CHILDREN: ● Children's Motrin Suspension or chewable tablets (over 2 years old) ● Infants' Motrin Concentrated Drops (6 months–2 years)

Belongs to a group of medicines known as non-steroidal anti-inflammatory drugs (NSAIDs). Widely used to treat muscle and joint pains, headaches, cold and flu symptoms (and fever), and menstrual cramps.

Method of use Usually, pills for adults. Liquid or chewable tablets babies and children. Take after food to minimize stomach irritation.

Side effects Usually mild; most likely problems are nausea and indigestion from pills.

Precautions Consult a doctor before using ibuprofen if you have or have had a peptic ulcer or asthma. Don't take if you have had an allergic reaction to ibuprofen, aspirin, or similar drugs, or a worsening of asthma or allergic symptoms. Don't give to babies under 6 months unless advised by a doctor. Discuss with your doctor before giving to children and babies. *See also* GENERAL CAUTIONS, p.176.

Insect bite and sting relief

Common brands
● Benadryl (diphenhydramine) ● Americaine Topical Anesthetic First Aid Ointment (benzocaine) ● Nupercainal Cream (dibucaine)

Contain an antihistamine (*see* p.178), such as diphenhydramine, to ease swelling and itching, or a local anesthetic, such as benzocaine. Can also relieve nettle or jellyfish stings. Hydrocortisone cream (*see* left) can be used for bites and stings.

Method of use Available as creams or ointments. Apply sparingly immediately.

Side effects Usually none. If rash occurs, stop using.

Precautions Don't apply to large areas, or to broken or sunburned skin.

Lactase supplements

Common brand
● Lactaid

May help people to overcome intolerance to milk or dairy products. Lactase helps to break down lactose sugar in the body so that it can be easily absorbed.

Method of use Take before eating or drinking dairy products.

Side effects Usually none.

Precautions See a doctor before use if you are diabetic or think a child has a food intolerance.

Lanolin ointment

Common brand
● Lansinoh

Creams containing lanolin protect skin and soothe and heal sore and cracked nipples in breast-feeding women. Use only medical-grade lanolin products.

Method of use Apply to nipples. Does not have to be wiped off before feeding baby.

Side effects Usually none.

Precautions None.

Lavender

Lavender (*Lavendula angustifolia*) is a traditional remedy that may help some people sleep.

Method of use Add essential oil to a warm bath or put drops on a tissue and inhale. Place sachets of dried lavender in a pillowcase.

Side effects Occasionally, skin irritation, nausea, and headache.

Precautions Don't use lavender essential oil if you are pregnant or breast-feeding. Never ingest essential oils.

Laxatives

Common brands
BULK FORMING FIBER SUPPLEMENTS: ● Citrucel (methylcellulose) ● Fibercon caplets (polycarbophil)
STIMULANT LAXATIVES: ● Ex-Lax (sennosides) ● Senokot (senna) ● Correctol (bisacodyl)

Laxatives relieve constipation. Bulk-forming types help stools retain water, making them softer, bulkier, and easier to pass. Stimulant types make bowel muscles contract and speed the passage of feces.

Method of use Fiber supplements as granules or powder, to be mixed with water and drunk; avoid taking at bedtime. Stimulant types are available as pills, powder, syrup, or as suppositories, normally taken at bedtime since they work overnight.

Side effects Mild bloating and flatulence withbulk forming types; mild abdominal discomfort just after taking stimulant types.

Precautions Drink plenty of fluids with fiber supplements. Don't use stimulant laxatives for more than 7 days at a time. Overuse may make bowels ineffective without them. Don't use if you have another digestive disorder. *See also* GENERAL CAUTIONS, p.176.

Lip creams, balms, and salves

Common brands
● Chapstick ● Blistex ● Neutrogena Lip Moisturizer ● Vaseline Intensive Care Lip Therapy

Moisturize and soothe sore, chapped, and cracked lips and mouth. Petroleum-based products protect against dryness in cold weather. Ski protection types have a sun protection factor (SPF) of 15 or higher for use at high altitudes.

Method of use Available as solid sticks, creams, ointments, or gels. Apply as needed.

Side effects Usually none.

Precautions Don't use on broken skin.

Lubricating jelly

Common brands
LUBRICANTS: ● Astroglide ● K–Y Lubricating Jelly
VAGINAL MOISTURIZER: ● Replens

Water-soluble lubricants applied to penis or vagina to ease dryness and soreness. Available as gels or vaginal moisturizers. Safe to use with condoms (unlike oil-based lubricants, such as petroleum jelly or baby oil, which can break down latex).

Method of use Apply to vaginal entrance or penis prior to intercourse; longer-lasting vaginal moisturizers applied internally several times a week to provide continuous moisture.

Side effects Usually none.

Precautions Don't use vaginal moisturizers during or just after pregnancy.

Migraine remedies

Common brands
● Excedrin Migraine (acetaminophen, aspirin, caffeine)

Relieves the pain of migraine headache.

Method of use Take 2 pills with a glass of water as soon as symptoms or aura begin to develop. Do not take more than 2 pills in 24 hours unless advised to do so by your doctor.

Side effects See acetaminophen (*see* p.177) and aspirin (*see* p.179).

Precautions While taking, limit intake of drinks containing caffeine. Too much caffeine may cause nervousness, irritability, and occasionally, palpitations. *See also* GENERAL CAUTIONS, p.176.

WARNING
Don't take remedies containing analgesics with other analgesics due to risk of overdose. Children and teenagers should not use this medication for chicken pox or flu syndromes before a doctor is consulted about Reye's syndrome, a rare but serious illness reported to be associated with aspirin.

Minoxidil

Common brands
● Rogaine Regular Strength (for men and women)
● Rogaine Extra Strength (men only).

May prevent hereditary hair loss or promote hair growth but must be used continuously to maintain effect. Works best on small areas in younger adults with recent hair loss. Extra-strength product available for more advanced hair loss. New growth may take a few months.

Method of use Usually applied twice a day to clean, dry hair and scalp using pump spray or roll-on applicator. Massage lightly into scalp. Wash hands after use. Don't exceed stated dose.

Side effects Brief scalp irritation; if it persists, stop using. Hair loss may increase slightly at first.

Precautions Avoid eyes and sensitive or broken skin. *See also* GENERAL CAUTIONS, p.176.

Moisturizers

UNBRANDED ITEMS: ● Water-based cream ● Emulsifying ointment

COMMON BRANDS: ● Lubriderm ● Curel Lotion ● Jergens Moisturizer

Wide range of moisturizers (emollients) to soothe, soften, and help the skin retain moisture. Preparations reduce dryness, itching, and scaling, and prevent cracking and infection in problems such as psoriasis and eczema.

Method of use Apply as often as needed, particularly after washing. Use water-based cream or emulsifying ointment instead of soap for washing.

Side effects Rarely, sensitivity to an ingredient; stop using and contact a doctor.

Precautions None.

Motion sickness pills

Common brands

● Dramamine (dimenhydrinate)
● Bonine (meclizine)
● Antivert (meclizine)

Help prevent motion sickness if taken before traveling. Products contain an antihistamine drug such as dimenhydrinate or meclizine.

Method of use Allow enough time for pills to take effect before you travel.

Side effects Some types may cause drowsiness, a dry mouth, or blurred vision.

Precautions Don't take with alcohol. If drowsy, don't drive or use hazardous machinery.

Mouth and throat treatments

Common brands

ANTISEPTICS: ● Listerine (thymol, eucalyptol, methylsalicylate, menthol)

LOCAL ANESTHETICS AND ANALGESICS: ● Dequacaine (benzocaine, dequalinium) ● Chloraseptic Sore Throat Lozenges (benzocaine, menthol) ● Chloraseptic Sore Throat Spray (phenol) ● Anbesol (benzocaine) ● Oragel Maximum Strength (benzocaine)

CLEANSING MOUTH WASHES: ● Lavoris ● Scope

BREATH FRESHENERS: ● Binaca Breath Spray ● Listerine Cool Mint Oral Care Strips Pocket Packs

Various treatments for mouth and throat problems, such as bad breath, sore throat, or mouth ulcers. Those containing an antiseptic help sore areas to heal and prevent further infections. Local anesthetics such as benzocaine help relieve the pain associated with sore throat or mouth ulcers. Fresheners give breath a pleasant smell temporarily.

Method of use Liquids used as a rinse or gargle; sprays or gels applied directly to sore areas. Throat lozenges and breath fresheners are sucked or dissolved on the tongue.

Side effects Occasionally, irritation and soreness. Stop using if persists.

Precautions Some products are not advised for children. Check package. Do not use products containing local anesthetics for more than 7 days unless directed to by your doctor or dentist. *See also* GENERAL CAUTIONS, p.176.

Oatmeal products

Common brand

● Aveeno cream/moisturizing lotion/body wash/foaming bath oil

Help to soothe itchy skin caused by irritating and inflamed skin conditions.

Method of use Available as bath oils or as creams or lotions applied directly to the skin. Lotions can be used instead of soap when washing. Add bath oils to a lukewarm bath; pat skin dry.

Side effects Usually none.

Precautions Oatmeal bath additives can make the bathtub slippery; be careful when getting in and out of the water.

Oil of cloves

Cloves (*Eugenia caryophyllata*) are traditionally used to relieve various problems, including toothache. Oil of cloves helps numb the tooth area.

Method of use Apply a few drops to cotton balls and place directly on tooth. Keep the oil off the tongue since it may burn a little.

Side effects Usually none.

Precautions None.

Oral rehydration solutions

Common brands
- Pedialyte (dextrose, electrolytes)
- Rehydralyte (dextrose, electrolytes)

Solutions that replace water, fluid, and salts lost from the body due to vomiting, diarrhea, or excessive sweating.

Method of use Available as ready-to-use solutions in a variety of flavors. Follow the directions carefully.

Side effects Usually none.

Precautions Don't use more than 48 hours after opening the bottle.

Peppermint oil

Helps relax the bowel muscle and relieve pain and bloating in irritable bowel syndrome.

Method of use Available as enteric-coated capsules, which are resistent to stomach acid, so that the peppermint oil is released into the bowel directly. Follow the directions carefully; usually, the capsules are taken about 30 minutes before a meal, 3 times a day.

Side effects Using peppermint oil may cause heartburn.

Phytoestrogens

Natural plant chemicals, usually found in soy-based foods, that have a similar (but weaker) effect on the body as the female hormone estrogen. Also found in flaxseed. May help reduce menopausal symptoms such as hot flashes.

Method of use Boost diet with soy beans, soy-based products, such as tofu or soy beans, and flaxseed bread.

Side effects Usually none if products are taken as part of a normal diet.

Precautions None.

Pinworm treatments

Common brands
- Pin X (pyrantel) • Reese's Pinworm Caplets (pyrantel)

Pyrantel works by paralyzing the worms, which are then passed in the stool.

Method of use For adults and children over 2, pyrantel is available as a pill or liquid to take by mouth. It is usually taken as a single dose and may need to be repeated after 2–3 weeks to completely clear the infection.

Side effects Not common, but can include stomach upset, stomach cramps, vomiting, and diarrhea.

Precautions Consult a doctor if a baby has pinworms. *See also* GENERAL CAUTIONS, p.176.

Salicylic acid

Common brands
- Clear Away Wart Remover • Compound W Liquid
- Dr. Scholl's Corn Removers • Premier Corn Cushions

Salicylic acid softens hardened skin, such as calluses and corns, and warts, making them easier to remove. Available as liquids, gels, or ointments.

Method of use Make sure area is clean and dry. Wart treatment can take up to 12 weeks.

Side effects May cause mild soreness when first applied. If severe, stop using.

Precautions Avoid surrounding skin, broken or inflamed skin, moles, birth marks, warts with hair. Don't use on the face or genitals. Consult a doctor before use if you have diabetes.

Saline nose drops

These contain a simple saline solution that moistens the lining of nasal passages and loosens thickened mucus, making it easier to clear nasal passages.

Method of use Blow your nose first. Apply a few drops into each nostril. Hold your head back for a few minutes so that the drops run inside your nose.

Side effects Usually none.

Precautions Throw unused drops away at end of treatment.

Saw palmetto

A traditional remedy for men's urinary problems made from berries of saw palmetto (*Serenoa repens*). May improve urine flow and bladder emptying in men with benign (noncancerous) prostate gland enlargement.

Method of use Extracts available as pills or capsules. Take as directed. May be several months before you notice an improvement.

Side effects Can cause stomach upsets.

Precautions Discuss with a doctor first if you have symptoms of prostate enlargement.

St. John's wort

Preparations made from St. John's wort (*Hypericum perforatum*) are used as a remedy for mild depression. Some studies suggest they are as effective for mild depression as some prescription medicines but have fewer side effects.

Method of use Usually available as pills or capsules. It is advisable to consult a doctor first before treating yourself.

Side effects Headaches, anxiety, and skin sensitivity to sunlight.

Precautions Consult a doctor or pharmacist before use if you are taking any daily medication since St. John's wort can interact with many drugs. Don't use with antidepressants or birth control pills. *See also* GENERAL CAUTIONS, p.176.

Sunscreens and sunblocks

Products designed to protect skin from harmful ultraviolet (UV) rays in sunlight. Total sunblocks (containing zinc oxide or titanium dioxide) prevent all UV light from reaching your skin. Sunscreens are graded by sun protection factor (SPF); the higher the SPF, the greater the protection given.

Method of use A sunscreen with an SPF of at least 15 that protects against both UVA and UVB rays is recommended.

Side effects Some preparations may irritate the skin.

Precautions Don't use sunscreens or sunblocks on a baby under 6 months old.

Tea tree oil

Oil from the tea tree (*Melaleuca alternifolia*) traditionally used as an antiseptic. Tea tree products may be used to treat mild skin irritations and infections, such as cold sores.

Method of use Available as liquid that is applied to the skin.

Side effects May cause allergic skin reactions in some people; if affected, stop using.

Precautions Keep away from eyes, mouth, and sensitive skin.

Vitamin B$_6$ (pyridoxine)

Supplements of vitamin B$_6$, or boosting the diet with foods rich in the vitamin, may help prevent PMS, and also cyclical breast pain and/or lumpiness.

Method of use Available as capsules. May need to be taken for 2–3 months to benefit. Foods containing B$_6$ include poultry, fish, eggs, soy, oats, whole-grain products, bananas, and nuts.

Side effects Usually none.

Precautions Don't exceed the recommended dose of vitamin B$_6$; high doses may cause nerve damage.

Zinc lozenges

May shorten the duration of a cold if taken when symptoms first develop.

Method of use Take the lozenges at the start of a cold. Stop when it has gone.

Side effects May cause nausea and produce a bad taste in mouth.

Precautions None.

Zinc oxide cream

Commonly used to treat diaper rash. Forms a moisture-repellent barrier that protects the baby's skin from contact with urine.

Method of use Apply to clean, dry skin at each diaper change.

Side effects Usually none.

Precautions None.

Index

Acknowledgments

I am indebted to my wife Ann, a health visitor, for her unstinting support and encouragement and especially for her expert writing and contributions to the articles in the baby and child sections.

I would also like to thank friends and colleagues for their help and encouragement, especially Martin Dunitz, Josephine Lawson of the Josephine Lawson Physiotherapy Clinic, London, and Harry Ganz of The Garden Pharmacy, London. I would also like to thank Mr. David Abrams, Drs. Ian and Tanya Beider, Mr. Amir Kaisary, Irving Lancer, Dr. Fred Lim, Dr. Colin McDougall, Mr. Alan Naftalin, Menachem Salasnik, Dr. Lester Sireling, Dr. Richard Teller, and Dr. Bernard Valman.

Dorling Kindersley would like to thank:
Project photography: Gary Ombler
Additional photography: Peter Andersona, Jake Fitzjones, and Esther Ripley
Index: Hilary Bird
Proofreader: Alyson Lacewing
First aid validated by Dr. Vivian Armstrong

Models: Ann Baggaley, Babita Bholah, Angela Cameron, Steve Capon, Gary Harding, Karen Heaton, Rosalie Hunt, Jo Lyford, Shahid Mahmood, Freya Mahony, Charlotte Mahony, Tony Maine, Brian North, Benji Peters, Morgan Steel, Duncan Steel, Shelia Tait, Scott Totman, Jeremy Wallis.

Picture Credits: (abbreviations key: t=top, r=right) The Ivy Press Ltd/Guy Ryecart **p.17**; Allergy-matters Ltd (www.allergymatters.com) **p.23**; Science Photo Library/ John Radcliffe Hospital (tr) **p.29**; Science Photo Library/Eamonn McNulty (tr) **p.32**; Science Photo Library/Biophoto Associates **p.33**; St. John's Institute of Dermatology **p.34**; Science Photo Library/Dr P. Marazzi (tr) **p.35**; Dr. D. A. Burns **p.38**; Dr. D. A. Burns (tr) **p.39**; Science Photo Library/CNRI **p.40**; Science Photo Library/Dr. P. Marazzi **p.42**; Science Photo Library (tr) **p.44**; Science Photo Library **p.48**; Science Photo Library/Dr. Chris Hale (tr) **p.50**; Science Photo Library/Sue Ford (tr) **p.59**; Science Photo Library/St. Bartholomew's Hospital (tr) **p.70**; Science Photo Library/Dr. P. Marazzi **p.71**; Getty Images/Vicky Kasala Productions **p.92**; Science Photo Library **p.95**; Science Photo Library/ Dr. P. Marazzi (tr) **p.98**; Nauticalia Ltd **p.100**; Photofusion/Clarissa Leahy **p.145**; Mother & Baby Picture Library/ EMAP **p.146**; Getty/Photodisc **p.147**; Meningitis Research Foundation **p.150**; Science Photo Library/Chris Priest (tr) **p.151**.

All other images © Dorling Kindersley.
For further information see: www.dkimages.com